Teaching
for Health
The Nurse as Health Educator

Lyn C. Coutts RGN SCM RSCN RNT BSc(SocSci) MMedSci
Nursing Adviser to the Scottish Health Education Group;
Honorary Fellow, Department of Nursing Studies,
University of Edinburgh, U.K.

Leslie K. Hardy RN BN MScNEd PhD
Associate Professor, The School of Nursing,
University of Lethbridge, Alberta, Canada

Churchill Livingstone

EDINBURGH LONDON MELBOURNE AND NEW YORK 1985

CHURCHILL LIVINGSTONE
Medical Division of Longman Group UK Limited

Distributed in the United States of America by Churchill Livingstone Inc., 1560 Broadway,
New York, N.Y. 10036, and by associated companies, branches and representatives
throughout the world.

First published 1985
   Reprinted 1986
   Reprinted 1987
   Reprinted 1989
   Reprinted 1990

ISBN 0-443-02751-X

British Library Cataloguing in Publication Data
Coutts, Lyn C.
   Teaching for health.
   1. Patient education   2. Nurse and patient
   I. Title   II. Hardy, Leslie K.
   613'.07   RT90

Library of Congress Cataloguing in Publication Data
Coutts, Lyn C.
   Teaching for health.
   Includes index.
   1. Nurse and patient.   2. Health-Study and teaching.
I. Hardy, Leslie K.   II. Title.
RT86.3.c68   1985   610.73   84–11365

Printed in Great Britain at The Bath Press, Avon

Parnys 3933 (1) $\int$11·50·391

5078

(Cou).

HJH P.

eaching
for Health
The Nurse as
Health Educator

3

98

B74216

Preface

In recent years much attention has been paid to education of the public about their health status. This text promotes the belief that the quality of life is directly related to the quality of health and that nurses have an integral role to play in teaching for health.

The phrase 'teaching for health' has been carefully and deliberately chosen. Ideas and thinking about health education have changed radically in the past few years, and there are wide ranging opinions on how health care professionals should go about the business of promoting health. We have chosen a teaching approach as suitable for nurses, but wanted to emphasise that the process of teaching should be interactive rather than proactive. So the book promotes teaching 'for' health, not 'about' health.

The content of this book is reflected in the title: *Teaching for Health*. One concept explored is about health and why 'good' health is desirable; another is about the process of teaching so that the nurse can purposefully help individuals to become aware of their health status and to develop the motivation to maintain a level of well-being which allows them to experience an informed, self-determined quality of life.

We have written this book with the British nurse in mind,

and have provided examples and statistics which relate to the health of people in Britain today. Chapters 1 to 5 develop information students need before they begin to teach. We have presented: a discussion on the concept 'health' and how one finds out about the health status of a population; a history of health education developments; aspects of the teaching and learning process; and the relationship of persuasion and communication. The last four chapters outline the process involved in teaching for health. Examples in nursing practice are used to emphasise how the ideas may be applied.

While the ideas in this book are directed towards improving nursing care, we also hope that students will evaluate themselves, their health status and their health priorites. Reference to the nurse as 'she' is used for consistency and is not meant to exclude the male members of the profession. Learning objectives begin each chapter as a guide to the students; further reading is indicated at the end of the chapters for those who wish to pursue the subject matter in depth and a knowledge review is included at the end of the book.

Good health to you!

Edinburgh and Lethbridge, Alberta, 1985   L.C.C.
                                                            L.K.H.

Acknowledgements

An essential feature of preparing for this book meant reviewing the literature in-depth and historically but, since health education promotes, reflects and involves change, it was also necessary and fun to discuss it with colleagues and friends. We owe a debt of gratitude to many people who provided stimulation and encouragement.

Special thanks are due to: Gail Ewing, whose doctoral research on stoma appliance management in the Department of Nursing Studies, University of Edinburgh, provided innovative ideas about self-care and teaching plans, some of which we have utilised; Olive Beaton who cheerfully accepted the task of deciphering our writing to type the rough drafts and manuscript; Jill Hughes, who, as a true friend, allowed us to ask of her some impossible tasks which she achieved.

L.C.C.
L.K.H.

Contents

Health promotion and the nurse

OBJECTIVES

Study of this chapter will enable you to:

1. Explore the meaning of health.
2. Identify current problems of ill health in Britain.
3. Distinguish types of statistics relating to the measurement of ill health.
4. Consider the concept of health promotion.
5. Discuss the ethical issues involved in health promotion.

WHAT DOES HEALTH MEAN?

Notice how the question is raised. Not 'What is health?', but what is meant by the term. Posing the question in this way acknowledges that health is not a fact, it is a concept. In a sense, what we are saying is that it is a matter of opinion what health is.

In the Judeo-Christian tradition health meant wholeness; it contained the idea of blessedness or salvation. Greek and Roman ideas on health centred on the concept of well-being. Health and happiness were closely related. Many modern definitions reflect synthesis of such ideas. It is often said that health has three dimensions which are in delicate balance: physical, mental and social. Some people indicate that there is a fourth dimension, that of spiritual health. Upset in any one of these areas affects the others. For instance, it is common to suffer a feeling of depression after viral infection. So there exists the idea that health is a state of balance between various aspects of life. When these aspects are in balance, we experience a quality of life we call health.

Katherine Mansfield (Savary et al, 1970) has described what that quality of life meant to her:

> By health I mean the power to live a full, adult, living, breathing life in close contact with what I love ... I want to be all that I am capable of becoming ...

This statement reflects the idea that health is dynamic; that being healthy has something to do with achieving potential. It also implies that health represents a condition of mastery in which the extent of growth and the direction of potential lie with the individual. Many people share such a view. It is commonly claimed that the purpose of being healthy is to be able to live well, on one's own terms. To decide on the meaning of health, then, is to make a value judgement.

Individuals define health on the basis of assumptions they make about the purpose and value of being healthy. Some assumptions which may be made about health are illustrated in Table 1.1. Clearly such a list could be extended considerably. Health has some elusive qualities which make it difficult to define. Also people have differing interpretations and aspirations. This creates a complex situation in which it is difficult to establish criteria to be considered in arriving at a definition of health. Is social conformity an important aspect? Are criminals healthy people? Which is more important: emotional satisfaction or physical fitness? Some individuals appear

Table 1.1 Some assumptions about health: Adapted from *Health Education and the Nurse* National Nursing and Midwifery Consultative Committee, Scotland, 1983, published by the Scottish Home and Health Department.

Health means different things to different people.
Health means more than the absence of disease or infirmity.
Health equals adaptability.
Health optimum varies.
Health is necessary for the purposes of life and adds to the quality of life.

to be obsessed with their health. Are they more healthy than others? Is sensible control preferable to obsession? What is sensible control?

Professional statements about health are also value judgements, based upon the goals and beliefs of the profession concerned. For instance, school teachers may be inclined to see the purpose of being healthy as related to being able to be socially useful. This is because many teachers accept that the goal of the educational system is to prepare students for life in society. Similarly, health care professionals may assume that prevention of disease should command a prominent position in values related to health because they are convinced that absence of disease adds quality to life.

There is nothing wrong with either view. Indeed, it can be argued that the latter is a proper professional perspective for nurses since the prevention of disease and care of the diseased person justify their professional existence. What is important is that health care professionals are aware of the origins and the limitations of their ideas about health, and that they are sensitive to the fact that individuals may want to decide for themselves about life and health.

One way to guard against having a limited view of what it means to be healthy is to be open-minded in approach to people and to be aware that health is a matter of opinion rather than of fact. It may be helpful to remember particular instances to bring this discussion into the context of reality. Take the case of the 19 year-old male who has survived a car crash but who is now paraplegic. Weeks of rehabilitation have enabled him to go home in the care of his parents. He manages most of his daily living activities and he feels a responsibility which prompts him to self-help in areas of skin and catheter care. He has talked about never achieving his dream of becoming a heavy machinery operator and now is asking for career counselling about what he can do. Is this young man healthy?

PLANNING FOR HEALTH

It is part of every nurse's responsibilities to be involved in planning to maintain or improve the health of individuals or

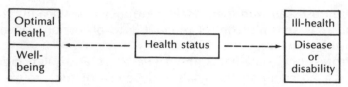

Figure 1.1 Continuum of health

communities. As well as being concerned with values, health is also a dynamic concept which means that the health status of an individual may vary with time, place and circumstance. For working purposes, the nurse may consider 'health status' as a moveable point on a continuum. Figure 1.1 illustrates a model of such a continuum. This model may be applied to communities as well as to individuals. An assumption that can be held about the model is that the extent and nature of ill health are neither predetermined nor a matter of chance and that it is possible to intervene to prevent deviation from 'normal' or average health in the direction of disease or disability and to facilitate movement towards optimal health. In other words, it is possible to plan for health.

Although optimal health and disease are at different ends of the continuum, it need not be assumed that there is a dichotomy of action between disease prevention and health promotion. In reality, what prevents disease promotes health and vice versa. Disease and health are interrelated. This text assumes that disease prevention is an integral part of health promotion.

Influencing the patterns of health in given communities is achieved in 5 main ways: environmental control, nutritional policy, immunisation, screening and health education. Strategies for health promotion require the application of a range of fiscal, legal and social controls. Such strategies have to be widely based. The promotion of health is not the exclusive responsibility of health care professionals. A variety of agencies are involved: education, employment, housing, transport and social services, as well as individuals themselves.

Three terms have been used traditionally in relation to strategies for the prevention of disease:

Primary prevention: action to prevent disease or disability before it occurs

Secondary prevention: action related to early detection and treatment of disease

Tertiary prevention: action to avoid needless progression or complications of disease.

Examples of such strategies are given in Table 1.2. Note that the activities described as primary prevention are very much concerned with health promotion. A comprehensive programme of prevention directed at any specific disease may incorporate all three aspects. In alcoholism programmes, primary prevention may be concerned with influencing mores about social drinking, while secondary prevention attempts to identify individuals in early stages before the addiction is established, and tertiary prevention is directed at minimising the effects of alcoholism, for example by maintaining good nutrition and therefore limiting harm to the liver.

Table 1.2 Examples of the strategies for prevention

Primary prevention	Secondary prevention	Tertiary prevention
— immunisation — provision of clean water — control of air pollution fluoridation of water supplies — car seat belt legislation	— eyesight screening in schools — deafness screening in certain occupations — breast self-examination	— checking for complications in diabetes mellitus — preventing damaging fits in epilepsy — limitation of joint damage in rheumatic conditions

The nurse involved with health promotion strategies must have a scientific basis for her plan. This means she must gather and interpret available health and vital statistics. The classic approach to health promotion employs the skills and insights of the epidemiologist.

Epidemiology is usually defined as the study of the determinants of the incidence[1] and the prevalence[2] of disease. The

Note: The terms 'incidence' and 'prevalence' have specific meaning. Often the words are used loosely as a general description of frequency. The precise definitions are:
1. Incidence—the number of new cases or events occurring per unit of the population at risk per unit of time.
2. Prevalence—the total number of cases identified per unit of population at risk per unit of time.

epidemiologist collects data relating to the distribution and size of disease problems. By examining the data it is often possible to identify factors contributing to disease patterns. Nowadays, it is increasingly realised that the epidemiological method may also be utilised to record patterns of health-related behaviour.

Knowledge of the size of a disease problem and of the behavioural and other factors contributing to that problem allows for planning of services, both curative and preventive. The epidemiological approach to planning is to seek to answer a series of questions:

— is there a problem?
— how big is it?
— how serious is it?
— is it amenable to influence by educational method or environmental engineering?
— will the costs be justified?

MEASURING HEALTH

Health professionals are expected to demonstrate that their work is effective in improving health, and for this, measurements are needed. If health is described in a way which allows measurement, then it should be possible to assess the current state of health of either an individual or a community and to set goals for maintenance or improvement. Measurable goals will also allow for evaluation.

Finding measurable aspects of a concept as elusive as health has proved problematic. In 1947, the World Health Organization (WHO) defined health as:

> a state of complete physical, mental and social well-being and not merely the absence of disease and infirmity.

It is impossible to demonstrate the achievement of such a goal. The difficulty is related to the problem of measurement. What is well-being? Exactly what does the individual have to feel or be able to do to be described as 'well'? Attempts have been made to distinguish levels of wellness and have been described (Galli, 1978). However, gaining agreement on the value to place on the various aspects considered to comprise wellness has proved, so far, an insurmountable task. The solution to this problem has been to use negative indices of health, mainly in the form of *mortality* and *morbidity* statistics.

Mortality statistics

These are available from the records kept under current requirements laid down in the Births and Deaths Registration Act of 1968. In Britain, births and deaths have had to be registered since 1836. When deaths are registered, the cause of death is recorded along with age, sex and social class. This means that figures from which to compile statistics relating to death rates from the various causes in different ages and social classes are readily available. Moreover, since the records have been kept for some time now, it is possible to study trends in the pattern of diseases.

Morbidity statistics

These record the amount of illness in a community. There are many parameters, for example, general practitioner consultations, sickness absence, hospital admission and reports of illness surveys. Morbidity data are less readily available at national level than mortality figures. Survey data about illness are often generated within research projects which look specifically at one disease or group of diseases, and consequently the available picture is somewhat patchy. A regular source of information is provided by the General Household Survey (GHS) which is conducted annually with a sample size of 30 000 persons. This is a multi-purpose household survey of Great Britain which has been carried out since 1971. The health section of the survey collects data on general practitioner consultations, outpatient visits and acute and long-standing illness. The data depend, of course, upon the self-reports of the people interviewed, and are subject therefore to the vagaries of perception and memory. This makes them difficult to interpret. Other sources of morbidity data are figures relating to sickness absence and hospitalisation and the national surveys of general practice consultations, the second of which was done in the year 1970–71. A comprehensive account of sources of mortality and morbidity statistics is given in the Central Statistical Office (1982) guide to official statistics.

The existence of reasonably accurate morbidity and mortality statistics allows the determination of the extent of disease problems in given populations. They can also be utilised to establish the seriousness of any problem and the scope for prevention.

Population statistics

To make sense of data relating to health, it is necessary to have some background information relating to the size of the population under study and its composition in terms of such factors as age, sex and social class. The main sources of such information in Britain today are data gathered during the *Census* which is carried out at 10-yearly intervals. This began in 1801 and was missed only once, in 1941, during the Second World War. The Census provides information on numbers of persons, age, sex, occupation, nationality, residence and type of housing. Questions covering certain additional topics are sometimes included. The Office of Population Censuses and Surveys is the Government agency responsible for arranging the Census and analysing the data. Further statistics are provided from data gathered because of the *registration of births* and because marriages, divorces and abortions are also required, by law, to be registered.

Epidemiologists gather data from the Census and registrations to draw a profile of population characteristics and trends. Health-related statistics, such as morbidity, mortality and use of services figures, are collected in order to be able to determine the frequency of a disease or an ill-health problem or health-related behaviour, and are often expressed as rates rather than as crude figures. Using rates helps to determine the size of a problem. Clearly it is not much use to be able to say that 100 people have died of a disease. That reveals nothing about the size and seriousness of the problem. Does it mean 100 people out of 100 died, or 100 out of the U.K. population? Are these the only recorded cases this century, this year, or this week?

Using rates avoids these difficulties, because a rate refers to the number of events recorded in relation to the population at risk over a specified period of time. There are three types of rates: crude rates, adjusted (or standardised) rates and specific rates. Crude rates are expressed in terms of a total population. There are limitations to this, as not everyone in the population shares the same risks. To avoid these limitations, adjusted or specific rates are used. Table 1.3 shows rates which are commonly referred to in assessing the health status of different populations.

Table 1.3 Common rates used in assessing the health status of populations

Name	Event	Population at risk
Crude death rate	deaths	total population
Birth rate	births	total population
Fertility rate	births	females 15–44/49
Stillbirth rate	still births	total births (live and still)
Infant mortality	deaths under 1 year	live births
Neonatal mortality	deaths under 1 month	live births
Perinatal mortality	deaths under 1 week and still births	total births (live and still)

In some ways, examination of the mortality statistics gives the most accurate picture of the pattern of disease in a community. Some distortions of these rates do occur due to difficulties in diagnosis, changes in disease classification, or to selective avoidance of diagnosis by doctors, but it is generally agreed that the cause of death recorded at present in the United Kingdom and other Westernised societies is reliable. A limitation of mortality statistics is that they give no idea of the nature of the ill health problem nor of its impact on society. Morbidity statistics, on the other hand, allow us to consider the amount of ill health which exists and to estimate its social and treatment costs.

As mortality and morbidity statistics are negative indices of health, it must be remembered that to assess the health of a community solely on the basis of such information is to miss something of the essence of health. Nevertheless, this is the only reliable information currently available on which to base plans for health. The prevention of disease is not the last word in health promotion, but it can be argued that it provides a necessary first step.

CURRENT ILL HEALTH IN BRITAIN

Mortality

The pattern of ill health in Britain has changed drastically since the turn of the century. For a start, most people live longer. 75% of all deaths occur at age 65 and over (Office of Population Censuses and Surveys, 1978). In 1901, life expectancy at birth was 48 years for males and 51 years for females. More recent calculations indicate that the life expectancy at birth is 70 years for males and 76 years for females (Central Statistical Office, 1983). In the 19th century the main causes of mortality, once the hazards of birth were surmounted, were infectious diseases such as scarlet fever, measles, whooping cough, diphtheria, typhoid fever, cholera, tuberculosis and smallpox. In the 100 years from 1875 till the mid 1970s death rates from these diseases had been reduced by 99%. Over the past 30 years there have been dramatic falls in the incidence of infectious diseases. Diphtheria and acute poliomyelitis have been virtually eradicated, and tuberculosis, though still present, no longer makes an important contribution to mortality rates. Some infectious diseases do occur still: 1978 brought the worst epidemic of whooping cough since 1957, and the incidence of measles fluctuates considerably. However, the major threats to life today are chronic degenerative diseases rather than acute infections (DHSS, 1976).

The current main causes of death in Britain are heart disease, cancer and stroke, in that order. Other major causes of death are accidents, violence and respiratory diseases. Between them, circulatory diseases, neoplasms and accidents now account for 75% of all deaths (Office of Population Censuses and Surveys, 1978). Between the ages of 15 and 64 the single most frequent cause of death for men is ischaemic heart disease, with cancer, especially lung cancer, a close second. For women, cancer, especially breast cancer, is the most frequent cause of death, though circulatory diseases also make an important contribution to female deaths.

In the first year of life, respiratory diseases are the most prominent cause of death, followed by congenital abnormalities, 'sudden' deaths, infectious diseases and accidents. Between the ages of 1 and 35 deaths are few, and in the main are due to accidents rather than to disease. Common causes of death in this age group are suffocation in the very young, injury due to fires in the 5–14 year olds, and poisoning in those over 15 years. In people over 65 years old the greatest number of deaths are accounted for by circulatory disease, but respiratory disease, cancer, accidents and violence also contribute (Registrar General Scotland, 1983; Office of Population Censuses and Surveys, 1983).

Though babies born in Britain now have a better life expectancy than those born at the turn of the century, there are some individual differences worth noting. Firstly, girls fare better than boys.

Male mortality rates exceed female mortality at each stage in the life span, and this has been the case since records were first kept. The net result is a preponderance of females in the elderly population. More importantly, the widespread premature death of either sex means increasing numbers of elderly people have to adjust to living alone for extended periods of time.

Secondly, some groups in the population are likely to live longer than others. There are regional variations in age specific mortality rates, so that at present, someone living in the South East of England has a better chance of reaching retirement age than someone living in Wales or the North (DHSS, 1980). This is a fairly recent phenomenon: in the 19th century the South East of England recorded high death rates, whilst the far North was a much healthier place to live. As well as regional variations in mortality there are differences related to social class.

For the purposes of analysing health statistics, the most frequently applied categorisation of social class is the one used by the Registrar General. This categorises people according to occupation. Since 1970 the classification used has been as follows:

Class Occupational category

I	Professional (e.g. accountant, doctor, lawyer)
II	Intermediate (e.g. manager, school teacher, nurse)
IIIn	Skilled non-manual (e.g. clerical worker, secretary, shop assistant)

IIIm   Skilled manual (e.g. bus driver, butcher, coal-face worker, carpenter)

IV   Partly skilled (e.g. agricultural worker, bus conductor, postman)

V   Unskilled (e.g. labourer, cleaner, dock worker)

5% of the population fall into Class I, 18% into Class II, 12% are Class IIIn, 38% Class IIIm, 18% Class IV and 9% are in Class V.

A recent report of the DHSS (1980) revealed that a child born to parents in Class I, provided he does not change his class, is likely to live 5 years longer than a child born to parents in Class V. Class differences in mortality persist throughout the human lifespan, with mortality tending to rise inversely with falling status. The babies and children of unskilled manual workers are less likely to survive their first year than those of professionals. Twice as many babies of Class V die within the first month, and between one and 12 months 4 times as many girls and 5 times as many boys die. The risk of death from fire, falls or drowning between 1 and 14 years is ten times higher for boys in Class V than in Class I.

Class differences in mortality are less marked for adults, but a class 'gradient' in favour of the upper classes can be demonstrated for many, though by no means all, causes of death. Class is significant for both sexes in infectious and parasitic diseases, blood diseases and diseases of the respiratory and genito-urinary systems. There are steep class gradients for women in circulatory disease and in endocrine, nutritional and metabolic diseases and for men in malignant neoplasms, accidents and diseases of the nervous system (DHSS, 1980).

Occupation, as categorised by the Registrar General, provides a very crude tool with which to judge social class, and one which may need refining. Income, property, education and housing tenure have been proposed as alternative variables which might be used to stratify the population (DHSS, 1980). Nonetheless, even this crude tool generates such consistent results that there can be little doubt that there are real inequalities of health in Britain today, at least on the basis of existing mortality statistics.

Morbidity

The available morbidity statistics provide further interesting information about the state of the nation's health. Cardiovascular disease and cancer may be the greatest killer diseases of modern times, but dental caries is by far and away the most prevalent disease. In the past decade, dental health surveys in England and Wales have shown that at least 60% of children in all age groups to 14 years had active dental decay, and that the proportion was as high as 78% at age 8 (Todd, 1973). 39% of Scots and 28% of the English over 16 years have no natural teeth. The figure varies with age: 10% of Scots (3% of the English) between 25–34 years have no teeth, but the figure rises to 85% in the population aged 65 years and over (78% in England and Wales) (Todd et al, 1978). Morbidity statistics from general practice (Royal College of General Practitioners et al, 1979) reveal that the common causes for consulting a doctor are related to respiratory disease, with the common cold, tonsillitis and bronchitis featuring largely. Consultations for rheumatism and arthritis also take up a large part of the general practitioner's time as do mental disorders, particularly anxiety and depressive neuroses in females.

HEALTH EDUCATION AND HEALTH PROMOTION

Examination of the ill health in society today reveals quite clearly that many of today's problems could be prevented. Some diseases have their origins in the behaviour of individuals, in the things they eat or the leisure patterns they choose. Other factors governing ill health are not within the individual's control but are deeply embedded in the value system, organisations and structures of society. The responsibility for his health lies first, but not completely, with each individual. There are also collective and expert responsibilities. The present dominance of preventable diseases demands intervention. Nurses have a part to play. They have the same individual and collective responsibilities as other members of society. In addition, they have the expert's responsibility to help others become aware of health-related issues and responsibilities. That is where health promotion and the nurse's role unite.

Earlier, health was presented as a moveable point on a continuum. The health status of individuals or of communities may be influenced by a planned strategy directed at health promotion. One of the five main ways of influencing the health of a community is health education, which is a planned process aimed at helping individuals and communities achieve and maintain a level of health which is appropriate for them. Many different types of activity are labelled 'health education'. For this reason the term may be considered as an umbrella which encompasses a number of activities concerned with promoting the health of both the well and the sick.

Some of the main types of health education activities are:

1. community health education programmes directed by health education officers,
2. health promotion by the media,
3. education of patients, conducted by nurses and doctors,
4. schools' health education programmes, carried out by teachers,
5. self-help relating to health information and health care, enabled by voluntary groups, community workers or health care professionals.

Generally speaking, the purpose is to promote health. Since health means different things to different people, there are many definitions of health education, and a wide range of goals. The most commonly expressed goals have been summarised (Levin, 1977, p. 632). These are to:

1. Contribute to self-fulfilment of individuals and promote their well-being as individuals define (this);
2. Enhance the ability of people to cope effectively with health promotion, health maintenance and illness control;
3. Reduce undesired risks of disease and illness;
4. Help people maintain personal and civil integrity while receiving health care; and
5. Create more active individual and community participation in the health system by increasing, (a) personal competence in self-care, and (b) social skills in working within the formal health system.

Nurses are involved as health educators both in the hospital and in the community. Figure 1.2 shows community and patient education as part of a spectrum of activity directed at the

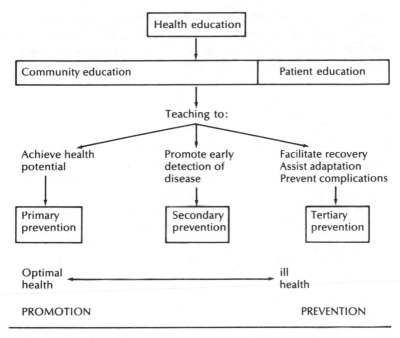

Figure 1.2   The relationship of health education and health promotion

continuum of health. Community education is channelled to the 'healthy' population: those who feel well, who have neither symptoms nor clinical signs of disease. It takes many forms: teaching school children about fluoride, advising antenatal parents, running weight loss classes, instructing in breast self-examination and so on. Patient education is intended for the person undergoing diagnosis, therapy or rehabilitation. Examples are: lessons on stoma management given to the person with a colostomy; instructions to a woman who has undergone hysterectomy about the limitation of activities; and discussion with someone scheduled for surgery about what to expect in the anaesthetic room.

Whatever the goals, a basic tenet of all health education is, first, that personal or collective behaviour influences health status and, second, that it is possible to change the health-related behaviour of individuals or communities by planned purposeful activity. The concept of planned influence may appear to be at variance with the goal of helping people maintain personal and civil integrity. Problems do arise in practice and are resolved according to the ideological and ethical position of the individual health educator.

ETHICAL ISSUES IN HEALTH PROMOTION

Since the definition of health depends upon value judgement there are bound to be ethical issues related to health promotion. These present a number of challenges to health professionals.

It is widely accepted that every individual has the right to assume responsibility for his own health, to define it for himself and to live accordingly. The problem is that to live to the full is not always to survive best. Many ill health problems of today are related to lifestyle choices which favour the development of chronic degenerative diseases. When people consciously choose what to do about health they often disregard the evidence that there are risks involved in behaviours such as cigarette smoking, over-eating and drinking and driving. Such behaviour results in conditions which are costly in social and economic terms.

Occasionally people act in a way that is counter to good health because they do not know any better. However, that is becoming rare in Westernised society. Usually the facts are available, but are ignored. There are a number of possible reasons for this. One may be that the person concerned does not value wellness or lack of disease. A sticky sweet now may be more attractive than keeping one's teeth all one's life. Watching sport on TV may win over playing tennis or swimming, despite the promise of a more supple old age. Enjoyment of the present is more meaningful than consideration of a vague distant future. Another reason is that people may not make a conscious choice about health-related behaviour. They may acquire habits over the years as part of their socialisation. Some people slip into regular drinking of large amounts of alcohol because they have grown up with the idea and the role models. Others spend the weekend hill-walking, watching the speedway, sailing, enjoying TV, maintaining a hobby for exactly the same reason. Some lifestyles are absorbed rather than chosen. If a conscious choice is made, it need not be made on rational grounds. Knowing the calorific value of cream buns does not always help the individual to refrain from eating them, even when the goal is to lose weight.

Influencing the health status of those individuals or communities engaged in unhealthy behaviour may require a planned purposeful intervention and that may involve an element of persuasion. That presents a dilemma. The rights of the individual may be at odds with the needs of society. Health professionals have to resolve the issues of that dilemma in order to be involved in health promotion and to reduce the social and economic costs of illness and premature death.

One question which arises is the extent to which it is reasonable to limit personal freedom in order to improve the quality of health of a community. There is no easy answer to such a question. In exploring the issue it should be recognised that there is no such thing as absolute freedom. With any degree of freedom comes the responsibility of considering the effects of freedom on others. It is not unknown for personal freedom to be sacrificed to the common good; for instance, the need for legislation to control road traffic is generally accepted and the need to have planning permission to extend property conceded.

Health educators are often asked to decide whether it is ethical to attempt to influence the choice of others. Some would argue that it is unethical not to. There is, after all, no values vacuum. It must be recognised that there are many persuasive agencies at work in a free society. Many of these offer an anti-health message: some confectionery lines and the tobacco industries are examples. Moreover, the expenditure available for such campaigns usually swamps sums available for health promotion.

So that the idea of eradication or limitation of disease for the common good may be invoked it is necessary to justify health education intended to persuade. In line with such justification it may be argued that nurses and doctors not only have a right but a duty to persuade others of the value of action to prevent disease. But does the professional duty to persuade conflict with a personal right to refuse to be involved in certain kinds of persuasion? What about the individual nurse whose ideas about respect for others make it difficult for her to accept the notion of influencing attitudes and manipulating lifestyle? Or the nurse who rejects the responsibility to be a role model?

It can also be argued for health education that, at the very least, individuals have a right to know what will affect their health. The persuasion issue can thus be avoided by assuming that all the health educator needs to do is present the facts about health without bias. But can bias be avoided? In itself, the decision to attempt to prevent disease introduces bias. Achieving a value-free presentation of facts may be more difficult than first appears. And what of individuals who declare that they want to live free from worry, and who consider that they have a right not to know what is harmful to their health? Some of the ways in which health educators respond to these ethical issues are described in Chapter 2.

REFERENCES

Central Statistical Office 1982 Guide to official statistics No 4. HMSO, London
Central Statistical Office 1983 Social trends 13. HMSO, London
DHSS 1976 Everybody's business. HMSO, London
DHSS 1980 Inequalities in health: report of a research working group (The Black Report). DHSS, London
Galli N 1978 Foundations and principles of health education. John Wiley & Sons, London
Levin L S 1977 Health education: moving to centre stage. Connecticut Medicine 39(10): 631–634
Office of Population Censuses and Surveys 1978 Trends in mortality 1951–1975. Series DH1 No 3. HMSO, London
Office of Population Censuses and Surveys 1983 Mortality statistics Cause 1982. Series DH2 No 89. HMSO, London
Registrar General Scotland 1983 Annual report. Edinburgh
Royal College of General Practitioners, Office of Population Censuses and Surveys, DHSS 1979 Morbidity statistics from general practice 1971–72. Second national study. Studies on medical and population subjects No 36. HMSO, London
Savary L M, O'Connor T J, Cullen R M, Plummer D M 1970 Listen to love. Regina Press, New York
Todd J E 1973 Children's dental health in England and Wales. Office of Population Censuses and Surveys Social Survey division. HMSO, London
Todd J E, Walker A M, Dodd P 1978 Adult dental health vol 2. Office of Population Censuses and Surveys Social Survey division. HMSO, London
WHO 1947 Constitution of the WHO. Chronicle of the WHO 1:3

FURTHER READING

Morris J N 1971 Uses of epidemiology, 3rd edn. Churchill Livingstone, Edinburgh
Murray R B, Zentner J P 1979 Nursing concepts for health promotion, 2nd edn. Prentice Hall, Englewood Cliffs, New Jersey
Thompson I E, Melia K M, Boyd K M 1983 Nursing ethics. Churchill Livingstone, Edinburgh
Wilson M 1975 Health is for people. Dartmann Longman Todd, London
Wilson R N 1970 The sociology of health: an introduction. Random House, New York

Concepts and styles of
  health education
Health education
  services in the United
  Kingdom

Nurses as health
educators
Teaching for health

2

Health education concepts and practice

OBJECTIVES

Study of this chapter will enable you to:

1. Discuss the various forms and guiding philosophies of health education practice.
2. Outline significant developments in health education during the past 100 years.
3. Describe the work of local and national health education agencies.
4. Discuss the role and function of health education specialists.
5. Describe how the nurse's role in health education has been variously interpreted and executed.
6. Consider the term 'teaching for health.'

CONCEPTS AND STYLES OF HEALTH EDUCATION

All health education has been and is based upon the assumption that the health status of individuals or communities may be influenced purposefully. However, opinions differ about how such influence can and should be achieved, and so the nature of health education varies with the underlying health aspirations of the society in which the health education takes place, the knowledge base and resources available to health educators and the assumptions which are made about the purpose of health education.

Health educators have been described as splitting into two groups: those who assume that they have a duty to use persuasive strategies to help people learn new patterns of behaviour, and those who assume that health education is aimed at assisting rather than persuading people to change (Simonds, 1977; Tones, 1977). It may be that these two positions are largely a reflection of differing beliefs of the teaching and medical professions (Vuori, 1980). Such a polarised distinction helps to identify one of the main ethical issues relating to health education, but clearly fails to deal with the complexity of the persuasion problem. Health educators are divided not only on the issue of whether or not to persuade. Opinions vary as to how persuasion is achieved, who needs to be persuaded and how persuasion should be applied. Health education is a multifaceted activity, employing a variety of means and strategies to deal with the promotion of health in society. A summary of how health education has developed in concept and practice over the last hundred years or so is presented in Table 2.1. Today, the main approaches, depending upon the style and purpose of the health educator, are information-giving, education, propagandising, enabling strategies and political action.

Information-giving

The information-giving approach includes such health education activities as preparing a leaflet, giving a talk, displaying a poster or producing a television documentary. The stress is upon presenting factual information in a way that makes it interesting and easily understood. Health educators who use information-giving strategies assume that it is their job to present people with facts about health and let them decide for themselves what to think and do about it. This assumes that people make conscious choices about health behaviour and that factual information will influence those choices; in other words, that man behaves rationally in relation to his health. Clearly, such an assumption may be challenged. It is true that

Table 2.1 Trends in the development of health education concept and practice

Underlying health aspirations	Prevailing purposes	Scientific bases emphasised	Methods in use
1850–1950 (approximately):			
Reduce infectious diseases, improve standards of hygiene, nutrition	Inform about health hazards, propagandise about the benefits of prevention	Medical science	Leaflets Posters Talks Blackboard Films
1950s–1970s:			
Prevent, cope with chronic disease	Acknowledge social aspects of health, help people take informed decisions about health options	Behavioural science	As above, plus sophisticated audio visual aids, groupwork, decision-making/problem solving, advertising, use of TV
Late 1970s onwards:			
Shifting emphasis from medical domination to lay participation in care	Enable participation in health care, acknowledge alternative forms of health care	Firmer adherence to both scientific bases, with emphasis upon making technical knowledge accessible and increasing concern about evaluation	As above, plus growing interest in non-directive techniques

some people make rational choices about health some of the time. However, the cigarette-smoking bronchitic and the nibbling weight-watcher provide just two reminders that rationality is not the only influence on health behaviour.

Another problem is that what appears rational to one person may appear irrational to another. For instance, it is rational to take time and trouble to care for one's teeth if one wants to keep them for a lifetime. It is equally rational not to spend energy, and perhaps money, on dental care if one believes dentures are an acceptable substitute for teeth. A serious limitation of the information-giving approach to health education is that it ignores the question of motivating people to adopt particular health-related behaviour. It assumes that everyone agrees about the meaning and purpose of being healthy and is anxious to achieve 'health'.

Doctors and nurses fall all too often into the trap of assuming either that their health values are generally held, or that, at the very least, lay people will acknowledge them as the right values since they are based upon professional knowledge and expertise. This undue emphasis upon rationality, coupled with the assumption that expert authority will be acknowledged, has led, until recently, to heavy reliance by nurses and doctors upon the information-giving approach to health education, and thus to use of the term *medical model* to describe this approach (Vuori, 1980; Thompson, 1983). Various models of health education are summarised in Table 2.2.

The origins of the medical model of health education lie in the 19th century, when the main health preoccupation was the control of infectious disease. A parallel concern was the interest of the great reformers in the welfare and social conditions of the working poor. The latter half of the century saw a rapid increase in the use of legislative power to improve living conditions generally and the lot of the poor in particular. It was a time of much social reform.

Many of the reformers were men of religion and aspiring to health was the Godly thing to do. Self-denial was a prominent theme, as is illustrated by the preface to a little book recording some health lectures given to the people of Edinburgh during the winter of 1880–1881 (Health, 1881) which states:

> The oldest record of man's history tells of a fall in condition from pure greediness of desire. God knows what was lost in early days, but the last, divinest teacher of the world struck again the keynote sounded by divine wisdom at Creation and declared that through self-denial alone we should reach not simply health but Immortal Life.

Such a social context set the scene for health educators to assume responsibility for telling people what to do and what not to do, since they operated in a society in which control of the many by a privileged few was usual. The time was also set for the emergence of doctors as the experts who could tell people about health.

Table 2.2 Models of health education

	Assumptions	Strategy	Tactics	Role of practitioner
Medical	The facts will persuade. The advice of experts is highly valued	Generate and promote clear and simple messages	Identify cost effective methods of presenting information. Package the material attractively	As expert informant, give talks, prepare booklets, exploit new media techniques to improve presentation
Educational	Education will elicit potential and achieve autonomy. Exploration of values and feelings will activate health action	Assess learning needs and readiness with reference to the group concerned and relevant research, then generate a systematic planned approach	Set clear objectives. Identify evaluation criteria. Ensure feedback	As educator/enabler, lead the person to learning discoveries, set up opportunities to discuss feelings and challenge 'facts'
Media	People have to be manipulated to value health and adopt a healthy lifestyle. Health can be 'sold'	Create and provide positive health images. Increase awareness of the impact of disease	Role modelling Repetition Rhetoric Fear arousal	As persuader, present an image and package the message persuasively
Community development	People have strengths. They will want to use them to improve their health on their terms	Offer a 'lets get together and talk about this' approach to determine felt needs	Organise discussion and communication among a wide range of individuals on given health issues to arrive at consensus	As enabler, help the person express discontents, encourage organisation to facilitate change, nourish interpersonal relationships
Political	Change in the institutions and structures of society is needed to improve health. Power, local and national, must be mobilised	Create an awareness of health issues. Influence the decision-makers	Lobby politicians, embarrass anti-health profiteers, mobilise local support	As provocateur, provide evidence, draft letters, facilitate action

Sanitary and other reforms of the 19th century brought gradual improvements in standards of living, including nutrition. Infectious diseases were combated and disease patterns changed. During this time medical and scientific discoveries accelerated and this led to an emphasis upon the contribution to health which might be expected from medical science. It seems to have been widely assumed that these new experts should process information for people and make judgements about health on their behalf.

As late as the 1960s in Britain, a report of the Central and Scottish Health Services Councils, known widely as the Cohen Report (Ministry of Health, 1964, p. 13), reflected medical domination over health matters in the statement that the 4 main contributions to health of health education were:

 (i) Advice about specific preventive measures
 (ii) Education with a view to inculcating habits and attitudes which will promote health and prevent disease
(iii) Education to understand the need for community health measures and support them
(iv) Education to seek advice from the doctor at an early stage for certain conditions.

The impact of the medical model was that health education developed as a tool of preventive medicine, concentrating upon the prevention of disease rather than emphasising the more positive aspects of health. Health education messages based upon the medical concept of being at risk of disease are often negative and threatening.

Education

The educational approach to health education challenges the naive assumptions of the medical model by acknowledging that beliefs, values and feelings may influence what people are prepared to do about health. This approach promotes the idea that the health educator should take the meaning of the term 'education' to heart, considering it as a means of leading toward discoveries rather than as a pushing in of facts. Because it adopts the rhetoric and methodology of educationists, this has been described as the *educational model* (Vuori, 1980; Thompson, 1983). The educational approach emphasises that health education should be concerned with affective (emotional) as well as cognitive (thinking) aspects of learning. It introduces the idea that each individual has a 'health learning career' (Tones, 1979) from the cradle to the grave, and proposes that health education activity should capitalise on the particular opportunities for motivating the individual which arise. For instance, the chance to shape attitudes of the child during primary socialisation or to change attitudes of the adult during life crises such as hospitalisation.

With this approach, much of the activity is directed at helping the person develop skills in decision-making and in clarifying thoughts and beliefs about health. A full range of educational methods may be employed, but often there is emphasis upon group work. The assumptions underlying the educational model have greatly influenced the development of patient education by nurses in the United States of America in particular. Redman (1978), for instance, has written about the advantages of a 'curriculum approach' to patient education. Recent publications relating to health education in British nursing practice have endorsed the educational model (Scottish Home and Health Department, 1983; Scottish Health Education Group, 1983).

Nonetheless, the model has limitations. The educational approach may provide an acceptable and successful way to change individuals. It does not, however, change the structures in society which perpetuate ill health. Although suitable for many nursing situations, particularly some types of patient education, if applied alone it may be too limited to effect sufficient change in health status differentials. Another limitation of the educational model is that it may bring individuals into conflict with existing value systems. For instance, children may question their parents' smoking. The approach needs a parallel support system and in practice this can be difficult to provide.

The educational model of health education evolved from the 1950s onwards out of growing recognition that health has social as well as medical aspects. When it was constituted in 1947, the World Health Organization (WHO) published its now well-known definition referring to health as 'not merely the absence of disease' (WHO, 1947). A few years later, the first report of an expert committee on health education of the public(WHO, 1954) acknowledged that:

> The first problem of concern to the community may not be directly related to health. It may be one of agriculture, transportation, irrigation, housing or accident prevention, or of mere subsistence. Co-operation for health begins with the problem of immediate interest, assists in its solution and then is ready to help on health problems as they become of serious concern to the community. (p.5)

This view that lay and professional priorities in relation to health might differ was coupled with the acknowledgement that health messages might be rejected unless they took account of the existing beliefs, attitudes and feelings of the people to whom they were directed. The report laid great stress upon how people learn, and presented health education as an activity planned to take account of the complexity of human learning:

> Health education, like general education, is concerned with change in the knowledge, feelings and behaviour of people. In its most usual form it concentrates on developing such health practices as are believed to bring about the best possible state of well-being. In order to be effective, its planning methods and procedures must take into consideration both the processes by which people acquire knowledge, change their feelings and modify their behaviour and the factors that influence such changes. (p.8)

In addition, it was emphasised that health education should be less concerned with 'information-giving' and 'publicity' and make more use of educational techniques and theories. Two types of educational method were distinguished: didactic methods, which assume that the learner is an empty vessel into which information is poured; and Socratic methods, which assume that people already possess information, feelings, interests and beliefs which will affect the learning process and which therefore have to be taken into account in planning health education.

Emphasis was laid upon Socratic, or 'two-way' methods and there was concern to ensure participation of people in the learning process, the rationale being that active learning is generally more effective than passive learning. There was also an assumption that involvement in the learning process would motivate the learner.

The nature of the educational model of health education which was promoted during the 1960s and 1970s is clearly reflected in statements made by Pisharoti (1975) about his understanding of the term health education. He described it as having 'knowledge, attitude and behaviour components' and being aimed at 'individual family and community behaviour and their interaction patterns'. He also stressed that health education was a 'process' and not a single procedure and that 'learning takes place through the efforts of learners', while the health educator 'provides the circumstances in which the learning takes place'. (p. 5)

Propagandising

The educational model assumption that the opportunity to explore information, values and feelings results in changed health-related behaviour is borne out for some of the population, but by no means all. The question of how to motivate change in health behaviour remained a concern throughout the 1960s and 1970s, despite increasing sophistication of health education planning and methodology. The educational model stresses the importance of developing the individual's skills in relation to recognising health options and making informed choices, but the tension between the desire to allow the individual the responsibility for his own decisions and the need to persuade him to act wisely, is reflected in this quote from a WHO (1969, p. 8) report on the planning and evaluation of health education:

> The focus of health education is on people and on action. In general, its aims are to persuade people to adopt and sustain healthful life practices, to use judiciously and wisely the health services available to them, and to take their own decisions, both individually and collectively, to improve their health status and environment.

The need to confront the problem of motivation has meant that there are always some people who argue that a propaganda approach to health education is necessary. This approach involves the use of poster campaigns and mass media for the purpose of persuasion. It assumes that the health educator knows best about health and has a duty to persuade others to adopt values and practices which are known to be beneficial in combating disease. Health educators who utilise propaganda argue that it is naive to assume the free choice of individuals in a society bombarded with anti-health messages. They claim that the individual should be persuaded to adopt good health practices for his own good and for the good of others. Propagandists typically concentrate upon ethical or emotional aspects of the argument and are less concerned about logic and the facts of the case. Because modern propagandising has made much use of television in particular, this approach may be referred to as a *media model* of health education. The media model assumes that there exists a mass and homogeneous audience of people and that 'health' may be marketed in very much the same way as other products. Clearly, both assumptions may be challenged.

Apart from the ethical issues it raises, propagandising is criticised by some health educators on the grounds that its effects are short-lived. Motivation springing from emotional response may not be maintained once the stimulus is removed. The impressive but short-lived successes of fear appeals in some 'stop smoking' TV programmes are an example.

Another limitation of the media model is that often, of necessity, it promotes simplistic messages about what are very complex health issues. Moreover, it is claimed that via the media model, health education may be powerfully, and even dishonestly, directed exclusively at the individual, placing an unreasonable share of the responsibility for health upon him without providing any support or reference system and thus contributing greatly to what has been described as 'blaming the victim' (WHO, 1981).

In more recent applications, the media model of health education has incorporated attempts by health educators to influence the presentation of health issues in such media outlets as women's magazines, soap operas, and the like, in addition to the traditional approach of advertising health images or messages.

Enabling strategies

The information-giving, propagandising and educational approaches to health education all, to a greater or lesser degree, assume that the responsibility for health education and the skills and resources needed for the process rest with professionals. Enabling strategies are based upon a different assumption: that people have strengths and abilities which they will be willing to contribute, on their own terms, to the process of learning about and achieving health.

By tradition, educators have often labelled themselves 'enablers'. It is part of the rhetoric of educationalists to describe themselves as working 'with' rather than 'on' people. So 'enabling' is an old idea in health education. It does, however, have some new connotations.

Since Illich (1971, 1974) questioned the wisdom of institutionalising both health and education, there has been growing concern about the 'medicalisation of life', in other words, about the extent to which health care experts generally, and doctors in particular, have influenced the interpretation of the term health (Kennedy, 1981; McKeown, 1976; Wilson, 1975).

The main thrust of these challenges is that health systems can no longer devote themselves exclusively to providing medical and paramedical care while ignoring all other influences upon health. The complex and costly health care systems of the Western world have been challenged as socially irrelevant and there is growing realisation that the optimising of health will depend upon achieving lay–professional partnerships in care and upon coordinating the activities of health workers with workers in the social and economic sectors.

An international conference held in Alma Ata, USSR, in September 1978 (WHO, 1978) declared it obvious that the 'health sector' would not achieve health by working alone and urged Governments to bring health care systems as close as possible to where people live and work, emphasising full and organised community participation. The conference proposed that traditionally separate levels of primary, secondary and tertiary care should be joined in a new approach in which the caring tasks and roles would be closely geared to needs as defined by the people themselves. For health education, the particular challenge is to move from thinking primarily about the prevention of disease, a medical bias, to the promotion of health based on people's needs.

In a paper outlining how health for all could be achieved in Europe (WHO, 1981, p. 1), the change was described thus:

> Health education has, in theory, gone far beyond an approach that seeks to improve health by changing individual behaviour without taking into account the environment which enables or reinforces the possibilities of such behaviour change. Health education has come a long way from just 'blaming the victim' to a concept of developing awareness of health and providing the opportunities for more informed choices. One of its main concepts is now that of the individual in health care as a competent actor in a community setting, rather than by passive compliance.

Recent initiatives in enabling strategies have sprung from a concern to deal with the economic and political realities of health and to address accusations that traditional health education approaches have only been effective with the middle classes. One such new approach to health education comes from the theoretical background of community development.

The community development idea holds out the hope that it will be possible to reduce factors which alienate large numbers of people in a modern industrialised society and to achieve a greater sense of community involvement. There are many ways of defining what is meant by community, but one approach is to accept that communities will be geographically determined and that everyone within a locality will be considered as belonging to the 'community', so that no state of 'them and us' can exist. Barriers, whether lay-professional or any other, thus disappear. The professional worker views all parts of the community as part of the client system and accepts that only goals which are mutually agreed may be pursued. Clients or patients are viewed as citizens who possess strengths and who are capable of participating in a problem-solving approach to achieving health.

The community development approach is new in health education. It is too early to say how health educators utilising a *community development model* (Hubley, 1978; Turner, 1982) may proceed and how they will be distinguished from those using an educational model. The main difference appears to be in the extent to which non-directive techniques are used. Community development is the very opposite of community provision, in which the health education service is provided on the basis of professional identification of needs. It thus challenges traditional approaches and complex professionally-devised health education planning models. Adherents of the community development approach claim that it offers the opportunity to improve human relationships, develops problem-solving skills and increases self-esteem in a way that will make health education relevant to multiply-deprived groups in society which are widely believed to have been failed by the traditional medical and educational models. The tactical and planning approaches of the educational model and the community development model are contrasted in Table 2.3.

Political action

The idea that there is a need for political activity to achieve societal improvements which will impinge upon the health status of individuals is not new. The practice of agitating for health is gaining new emphasis, however, and the role of health education in generating community action for health has taken on new dimensions in recent years. The purpose of community action is to stimulate communities to seek their rights, including their rights to health. The underlying assumption of the community action approach is that underprivileged communities cannot be expected to operate on their own behalf and require assistance to engage in conflict with powerful authorities. Given the inequalities in health which exist in Britain today (DHSS, 1980), it is increasingly likely that health educators will be challenged to be involved in political activity to help people achieve health. At the very least, some people will feel that health educators should play a part in bringing inconsistencies and inequalities in health care provision to the forefront for discussion. Others take the view that health educators should act as patient or client advocates, given the present unequal distribution of power in relation to health.

The exercise of political power to achieve health is a tradition stemming from the 19th century when many improvements in health were achieved by the exercise of legislative

Table 2.3 Contrasting approaches to health education practice

	Directive	*Non-directive*	
	Educator (at times with the help of the learner(s)	Group members	Enabler (often by asking questions)
Step 1	Identify and describe the target group	Some dissatisfaction or need for change felt but not expressed	Stimulate people to think what their health concerns/needs are
Step 2	Assess needs	Begin to be aware of needs	Stimulates thought about changes which would reduce concerns, meet needs
Step 3	Set objectives	Recognise specific changes needed	Stimulates people to consider what they could do to achieve changes
Step 4	Plan a teaching programme	In specific terms decide for or against trying to achieve changes or meet needs	If necessary helps people decide how to organise for the tasks they have decided to undertake
Step 5	Choose teaching methods and materials	Plan what to do and how to do it	Stimulates people as necessary to allocate tasks and decide on a timetable
Step 6	Carry out the teaching programme	Carry out the plan	Stimulates people to consider potential problems and plan avoiding action
Step 7	Evaluate	Assess what they have achieved and express their reactions	

power. Today fiscal and legal controls, such as taxation on alcohol and penalties for not using seat belts, are used as mechanisms to reduce the toll of modern ill health problems. Additionally, there is new emphasis upon the power of people in local communities (Kickbush, 1983) and upon the political role of the health educator in releasing such local potential. Recent WHO documents have spelled out inequalities in health and the need for governments to act to achieve health (WHO, 1978) and a *political model* of health education has been described (Thompson, 1983).

HEALTH EDUCATION SERVICES IN THE UNITED KINGDOM

Anyone who mentions backache or expresses the slightest interest in jogging or acupuncture, will be surrounded almost instantly by experts willing to advise on what to do and what to avoid. Ever since man first recognised that aspect of life we call health, there have been health educators, some amateur, some with more clearly defined status as experts or professionals.

Depending upon country and culture, the expert health educator may be a wise man, witch doctor, religious leader, health care professional, school teacher or union official. In Britain today, a variety of people consider themselves to be professional health educators. A health education service is provided for the sick as well as for the healthy and health education is carried out by a range of agents in a variety of places, but this text is limited to consideration of health education services within the National Health Service.

National organisations

The history of health education is as old as mankind, but it is only necessary to look as far back as the last century to trace the development of our modern health education service. At the end of the 19th century, and for the first half of the 20th, there was widespread belief that medical science would in time cure all ills and ensure the health of the population. Early health education services developed out of a desire to promote that belief and encourage people in the use of new services such as antenatal clinics. Local staff, often health visitors or public health doctors, prepared posters and exhibitions and gave public lectures to advertise the services.

By the 1920s it was realised that such *ad hoc* local arrangements were costly and duplicated efforts were wasteful. Sir Allen Daley, then the Medical Officer of Health for Bootle, in Lancashire, began to press for the formation of a central body to be responsible for the development of health education materials. He argued that a central body with good funding could coordinate efforts and do a great deal to promote the development of health education. In 1924 he presented a paper entitled 'The Organisation of Propaganda in the Interests of Public Health' to the annual meeting of the Society of Medical Officers of Health (Daley, 1959).

The paper aroused great interest in the idea of a central body and in health education generally, but some local authorities were worried that when accounts were audited, questions would be asked about spending money on health education. There were those who questioned whether or not it was legal to spend public money to persuade the public to adopt particular types of behaviour. A deputation went to Neville Chamberlain to convince him that there was need for legal support for health education. This subsequently was granted in Section 67 of the 1925 Public Health Act. Health education was now sanctioned in law and the movement towards a central organisation could proceed.

By 1927 the Central Council for Health Education had been constituted, with responsibility for developing health education in England and Wales. Twenty years later a parallel Scottish organisation was formed, the Scottish Council for Health Education. The Councils organised lecture tours, study days, exhibitions and health fairs. They also produced a wide range of audio-visual materials for use in health education and provided a back-up service for anyone, amateur or professional, concerned to develop health education services on a local basis.

The 1950s brought a series of reports on health education produced by the WHO (1954, 1958). These reflected growing awareness internationally of new challenges to health education, in particular the need to respond to the realisation that modern diseases arose from the very fabric of society and were inextricably linked with the lifestyle of individuals. There was growing appreciation that health education might be used as an instrument of planned social change, rather than merely as the information arm of preventive medicine.

One British response to these new challenges was to set up, in the 1960s, a Joint Committee of the Central and Scottish Health Services, with a remit to investigate health education needs and provision in the United Kingdom. The resulting Cohen Report (Ministry of Health, 1964) laid the basis for national and local health education services as they exist today. The Report recommended that there should be established, in England and Wales, a strong central body which would promote the development of health education, identify priorities and secure support from all possible sources, commercial and voluntary as well as medical, and assist local authorities and other agencies in the conduct of local programmes. Such a body would also be required to foster the training of specialist health educators, to promote the training in health education of doctors, nurses, teachers and dentists, and to evaluate the results of health education. A parallel body for Scotland was also recommended, which would absorb the health education functions of the Scottish Home and Health Department and the Scottish Council for Health Education.

Following the Cohen Report, two new central agencies for health education were formed in 1968. The Health Education Council took over the responsibilities for England and Wales previously exercised by the Central Council. In Scotland the new organisation, the Scottish Health Education Unit, operated in parallel with the Scottish Council for Health Education until they were both disbanded in 1980 at the formation of the Scottish Health Education Group.

The Health Education Council and the Scottish Health Education Group have very similar remits. In general, their activities include helping to determine health education priorities, mounting national campaigns, sponsoring research and surveys and producing health information and audio-visual materials. Both organisations act as centres of expertise, providing a source of epidemiological, sociological and psychological data for a wide variety of people involved in health education. They promote health education training for health care professionals, cooperate with local health and education authorities and maintain contacts with a wide range of voluntary organisations with a concern for health education.

Local services

The Cohen Report had recommended the establishment of local health education departments, but these did not come into being until after the reorganisation of the National Health Service in 1974, except for a number of notable exceptions in a few enlightened local authorities. At the reorganisation, the health education functions of local health authorities passed to the National Health Service, with the exception of some specialist areas like hygiene in food premises, which remained the responsibility of Environmental Health Departments in the local authority. Each health authority is expected to make specific provision for all the organisation of health education within its geographical boundaries.

At the time of the 1974 reorganisation of the National Health Service it was considered that most, though not all, health authorities would be large enough to justify the employment of a small team of specialists in health education. The idea of professionally prepared specialists in health education had been mooted in WHO Reports published during the 1950s (1954, 1958). These highlighted the tendency towards increasing sophistication in the approach of the health educator and the need for specialist preparation. The first of these reports (WHO, 1954) suggested that health authorities providing health education services would require to have at their disposal the services of qualified professional workers with special training and competence in health education. Until then, most health education had been in the hands of pioneers, often drawn from medicine and nursing, who had boundless enthusiasm but no additional professional preparation for the health education tasks they undertook.

The second report (WHO, 1958) described the role of the health education specialist. It was to be concerned with planning, organising, administering and evaluating health education services; giving guidance on the health education training of health workers, school teachers and others in relevant fields; giving assistance with the selection, development and use of educational methods and media; cooperating with others in research on health education problems and methods and providing consultation services for and assistance with running conferences, seminars and similar meetings concerned with health education. So the idea of the health education specialist was born and the way was paved for the development of locally based health education services, staffed by professionals with specialist preparation in health education. Growth of the speciality has been slow (Sutherland, 1979), but today there is steady expansion throughout the United Kingdom. In 1983 there were 430 of the new specialists (now called Health Education Officers) in England and Wales and some 43 in Scotland.

Tones (1977) has suggested that health education officers have particular expertise in the application of behavioural science to health and illness and that their activities should be threefold: provision of consultancy services in health and human behaviour; initiation and coordination of community health programmes; and action research into relevant client characteristics and evaluation of programme effectiveness.

Since 1974 there has been steady, if slow, growth in the establishment and development of Health Education Departments at local level. A typical local department is likely to consist of a Health Education Officer in charge of a team of health education specialists who may have been drawn from a variety of professional backgrounds. Sometimes this team of specialists has support from people with expertise in public relations or media and exhibition and display work. These departments provide both material and personal support for a variety of health educators working with both professional and voluntary agencies. Usually they are responsible for identifying local priorities in health education and will initiate new ventures.

NURSES AS HEALTH EDUCATORS

Nurses have taught people about health since the establishment of the profession. In the early days the teaching reflected the general concern about sanitation and living conditions. In her *Notes on Nursing* (1859), Florence Nightingale emphasised that ill health was the result of want of whitewashing and ventilation, as well as careless diet and dress. She proposed that the nurse should act as educator.

Nurses, like all other health educators, have a changing role in health education. Clearly, the nature of health education activity considered to be suitable will depend upon the environment in which nursing takes place and there will be many different interpretations of the term. Some nurses have described health teaching as a nursing tool, to be used to promote spiritual, mental and physical health. Others have gone further and suggested that the nature of nursing is such that teaching is of the very essence of nursing. Reviews of how the nurse's education role is perceived have been provided by Cohen (1981) and Redman (1980). These indicate that most nurses accept that they have a health education role, though there has been confusion over the extent and nature of the activity required and uncertainty about how the nurse's role complements or differs from that of the doctor's.

Perhaps one of the best known and most widely accepted statements on nursing is that prepared by Virginia Henderson (1960) for the International Council of Nurses in 1961. It describes the unique function of the nurse as that of assisting the individual, sick or well, in health-related activities he would perform unaided if he had the necessary strength, will or knowledge. That the nurse has a health education role is implicit in this statement. Moreover, she indicates something of the extent and nature of the role: the nurse assists the person to gain motivation as well as knowledge and skills and she directs her energies to the well population and to the sick.

Most nurses who write about the nurse as health teacher (see Redman, 1980; Narrow, 1979, for instance) indicate that the nurse's health education role arises as part of the usual process of nurse–patient interaction: the nurse reads cues which indicate to her the patient's readiness to learn and she responds to these by seizing or creating the opportunity for teaching. So that health education by nurses may be individually tailored to needs and delivery can be instantaneous. This view suggests that the skilled nurse will identify gaps in the patient's knowledge, sense how much information he wants, judge whether the patient is comfortable or relaxed enough to take in the information and gear her language and explanation to such factors as his social class, education and experience. She will also, if necessary, choose appropriate visual aids or written materials to augment verbal explanations.

The model of health education proposed is an educational one. The underlying assumption is that the nurse has special skills which she will exercise in assessing people's teaching needs, in planning and conducting appropriate teaching and in evaluating the outcome of her teaching plan.

In a recent British statement (General Nursing Council for Scotland, 1980) about the patient education skills required by Registered Nurses, the following were noted:

— identify the learning needs of patients and relatives;
— identify the learning opportunities available for individuals and/or groups in the clinical setting;

— select and use suitable teaching methods and materials;
— develop patient education within (a given) care setting;
— evaluate patient education programmes at a level which will allow for improvement of personal performance as a health teacher.

These statements reflect acceptance of the importance and complex nature of the modern health education role in nursing, as well as endorsement of the educational model.

The endorsement of the educational model of health education by nurses is further illustrated in a recent publication of the Scottish National Nursing and Midwifery Consultative Committee (Scottish Home and Health Department, 1983) which proposes that health education should be applied within the process of nursing to assist the individual to identify and take informed decisions about his health potential and health-related behaviour.

An important aspect of this Committee's report is that though it proposes that nurses should adopt a systematic approach to the planning and implementing of health education it counsels that such planning need not imply inflexibility nor the imposition of professional values. This is a crucial point to bear in mind at a time of rapid developments in health education. Of late there has been increasing emphasis upon the importance of actively involving patients in professionally provided health care. Health professionals have come to accept not only that the consumer ought to be involved in his own care, but that he has to be, and is, involved. The necessity arises in part from the nature of modern disease and treatment, today the clinician determining treatment faces not a single right course but a number of options, the choice of which is best made by doctor and patient together. It also springs from a greater wish on the consumer's part to be informed and to participate in care.

The concept of consumer participation is manifest in the movement which has been called self-care (Levin et al, 1977). The self-care concept assumes that the individual's integrity in making health decisions and his ability to perform on his own behalf take precedence over professional values. Self-care, therefore, means that patients may be involved in procedures previously carried out by medical and nursing staff and in taking responsibility for certain decisions about care.

Self-care means more than self-treatment, however. Health maintenance, disease prevention, self-diagnosis, self-medication and participation in professional care have also been identified as possible roles for the individual to adopt. Perhaps the most challenging aspect of the self-care concept is that it acknowledges that evaluation of care is based upon what the individual sees as relevant, not upon professional criteria of effectiveness.

Active participation of patients in their care will require some reweighting of professional and patient goals, with emphasis upon ending the domination of the professional and evolving new professional–lay relationships. In health education it will mean revising the idea that the health professional knows best. Levin (1978) has suggested that patient education in the United States has become institutionalised and inflexible, and that it is time to consider the adoption of at least a self-care perspective in health teaching. Patient education is not sufficiently established in Britain to suffer from institutionalising; nevertheless, it is clear that one of the important issues for nurses to tackle is how to evolve health education approaches which will meet these new demands for participation. There is obvious scope within daily nursing care for the development of teaching geared to participation. People may learn aspects of self-diagnosis, self-medication or self-treatment as they are allowed to participate in their care. Such learning may be supplemented by group instruction and use of visual aids or written materials. There are also the vitally important learning opportunities inherent in being able to join in decision-making and to undertake self-treatment under agreed and diminishing levels of professional supervision.

It seems likely, then, that nurses will adapt the traditional educational model of health education to fit such new demands. There may also be a case for considering that all five approaches outlined earlier have something to offer the nurse as health teacher. A recently published report on the health education in-service training needs of nurses (Scottish Health Education Group, 1983) has recorded the idea that no single model of health education may meet the variety of situations in which nurses operate. The report of a workshop which discussed the nurse's role in health education (Randell, 1982) reflects similar thinking.

TEACHING FOR HEALTH

Though health education varies in form and philosophy and nursing practice in health education will be similarly varied, this text has been entitled *Teaching for Health* on the assumption that the student of nursing is most likely to experience and practice health education based upon an educational model. The educational model of health education assumes that health behaviour is the result of learning and that it therefore can be influenced by an educational process in which the nurse assumes the role of teacher and the patient or client accepts the role of learner. In this text the process has been labelled 'teaching for health'.

Some nurses find it difficult to distinguish the teaching aspect of their work. Much of nursing is directed at assisting adaptation to the circumstances surrounding health and illness. Since learning is an essential part of adapting then it can be argued that all nursing is teaching. At the other extreme, some nurses may have a view of teaching based upon their own schooldays and see it as necessitating 'talk and chalk'.

This text is based upon the assumption that health teaching is an integral part of nursing and that it should be executed as a purposeful activity, using interactive teaching strategies which involve the learner in planning and evaluating his learning wherever possible.

In teaching for health, the nurse may help to identify and solve health-related problems by:

— informing
— advising
— helping with the acquisition of skills
— assisting with the process of clarifying beliefs, feelings and values
— enabling the adaptation of lifestyle
— promoting change in the structures and organisations which influence health status
— providing a model of values and behaviour related to health.

The last may present the individual nurse with a particularly difficult challenge. Most people hate to be viewed as exemplary. There is something unacceptable to many in the idea of setting themselves up as a good example. There is no easy answer to this. Patients and clients observe the nurse's behaviour and learn from it despite her intentions. This does offer an element of responsibility to the individual nurse. Perhaps what can be said is that each nurse has a right to be healthy and that her decisions about health should not be considered only in light of the impact upon patients or clients.

Every nurse has a right to decide for herself how she will give expression to her health teaching function. The approach she takes to teaching for health will no doubt reflect her philosophy of nursing and of life, as well as her beliefs about the nature and purpose of health education.

REFERENCES

Cohen S A 1981 Patient education: a review of the literature. Journal of Advanced Nursing (6): 11–16

Daley Sir Allen 1959 The central council for health education the first twenty-five years 1927–52. The Health Education Journal 17(1): 24–35

DHSS 1980 Inequalities in health: report of a research working group (The Black Report). DHSS, London

General Nursing Council for Scotland 1980 Guidelines on health education. General Nursing Council, Edinburgh

Health Lectures for the People 1881. MacNiven and Wallace, Edinburgh

Henderson V 1960 Basic principles of nursing care. International Council of Nurses. Basle, Switzerland. (reprinted 1970)

Hubley J 1978 Community education community development and health education. Community Education 1 Winter 78–79: 19–33

Illich I 1971 Deschooling society. Calder and Boyars, London

Illich I 1974 Medical nemesis: the expropriation of health. Calder and Boyars, London

Kennedy I 1981 The unmasking of medicine. George Allen and Unwin, London

Kickbush I 1983 Introducing the regional programme on health education and lifestyles. Community Medicine 5(1): 59–62

Levin L S 1978 Patient education and self-care: how do they differ? Nursing Outlook 26: 170–175

Levin L S, Katz A H, Holst E 1977 Self-care: lay initiatives in health. Croom Helm, London

McKeown T 1976 The role of medicine: dream mirage or nemesis. Rock Carling Lecture, Nuffield Provincial Hospitals Trust, London

Ministry of Health 1964 Report of a joint committee of the central and Scottish health services councils on health education (The Cohen Report). HMSO, London

Narrow B W 1979 Patient teaching in nursing practice: a patient and family centred approach. John Wiley and Sons, New York

Nightingale F 1859 Notes on nursing. Harrison and Sons. Reprinted 1980 Churchill Livingstone, Edinburgh

Pisharoti K A 1975 Guide to the integration of health education in environmental health programmes. WHO offset publication No 20. WHO, Geneva

Randell J 1982 Nurse tutors health education and the curriculum. Report of a workshop on health education in nursing held at Leamington Spa March 5–7. The Health Education Council, London

Redman B K 1978 Curriculum in patient education. American Journal of Nursing 78(8): 1363–1366

Redman B K 1980 The process of patient teaching in nursing, 4th edn. C V Mosby Company, St Louis

Scottish Home and Health Department 1983 Health education and nursing. A report by the national nursing and midwifery consultative committee. Scottish Home and Health Department, Edinburgh

Scottish Health Education Group 1983 Health education inservice training needs of district nurses health visitors and midwives. Scottish Health Education Group, Edinburgh

Simonds S K 1977 Health education today: issues and challenges. The Journal of School Health December: 584–593

Sutherland I 1979 Health education: perspectives and choices. George Allen and Unwin, London

Thompson I E 1983 Theoretical models of health education. In: Scottish Health Education Group. Health education in-service training needs of district nurses health visitors and midwives. Scottish Health Education Group, Edinburgh

Tones B K 1977 The role of the community health education specialist in the delivery of health care. The Health Education Journal 36(4): 106–133

Tones B K 1979 Socialisation health career and the health education of the school child. Journal of the Institute of Health Education 17(1): 22–28

Turner J 1982 Community development as an alternative strategy for health education. Unpublished seminar paper presented at the University of Edinburgh Department of Nursing Studies 27 January 1982. Mrs J Milburn (nee Turner) Argyll and Clyde Health Board, Health Education Department, Scotland

Vuori H 1980 The medical model and the objectives of health education. International Journal of Health Education (19): 12–18

Wilson M 1975 Health is for people. Dartmann Longman Todd, London

WHO 1947 Constitution of the WHO. Chronicle of the WHO 1 (3): 1

WHO 1954 Expert committee on health education of the public first report. Technical Report Series No 89 WHO, Geneva

WHO 1958 Report of an expert committee on training of health personnel in health education of the public. Technical Report Series No 156. WHO, Geneva

WHO 1969 Report of an expert committee on planning and evaluation of health education services. Technical Report Series No 409 WHO, Geneva

WHO 1978 Primary health care. Report of the International Conference on Primary Health Care. Alma Ata USSR 6–12 September WHO, Geneva

WHO 1981 Regional programme in health education and lifestyles. Regional Committee for Europe Thirty-first session, Berlin 15–19 September EUR/RC31/10 WHO, Copenhagen

FURTHER READING

O'Neill P 1983 Health crisis 2000. WHO Regional Office for Europe
  Copenhagen. William Heinneman Medical Books Limited, London
Thompson I E, Melia K M, Boyd K M 1983 Nursing ethics. Churchill
  Livingstone, Edinburgh
Williamson J, Danaher K 1978 Self-care in health. Croom Helm, London

3

Learning and teaching about health

OBJECTIVES

Study of this chapter will enable you to:

1. Identify the various activities which may be implied in the term teaching.
2. Describe the nature and extent of teaching as a nursing activity.
3. Demonstrate the complexity of human learning.
4. Discuss the concept of motivation in relation to human learning.
5. Identify the conditions which assist human beings to learn.
6. Discuss how teaching style may influence learning opportunities.

IDEAS ABOUT TEACHING AND LEARNING

To many people the word teaching conjures up a classroom, perhaps even a blackboard. A lot of teaching is done by telling, explaining, demonstrating and providing an example. In technologically advanced societies, teachers may amplify these activities by using audio-visual aids such as films, overhead projectors or working models. But sometimes teaching involves more than telling, explaining or showing people what to do. There are situations where it is possible to teach by allowing the person to find out for himself about the right thing to do or the best way to do it. So teaching can also be done by leading discussion, providing programmed learning texts or setting up other special learning experiences such as practice opportunities and workshops.

Defining teaching

The term 'teaching' encompasses a variety of activities. These include giving information or advice, counselling and helping people clarify their thinking, express their feelings, identify options or develop new skills. Teaching may be defined as the process of helping or enabling another person to learn. Some teaching is done deliberately according to a plan: school teachers teach spelling, driving instructors teach how to control the car, midwives teach about breast-feeding, and so on. Other teaching may not be deliberate: parents may teach their children how to smoke, school teachers may convince children that mathematics is important only for boys, doctors may teach patients to expect prescriptions. So there is unintended as well as intended teaching.

Defining learning

Learning is a basic human activity, essential to survival. Young children have to be protected from heat, cold, water and heights until they have learned about the dangers. People with limited learning capacity may never be able to live independent lives. The ability to learn helps us avoid danger, communicate with others, adapt to changed circumstances, earn a living, or enjoy the finer aspects of any art form. Learning may be conscious or unconscious, easy or difficult, painful or pleasant. Much of the time learning is taken for granted. But what is involved in learning?

Psychologists say learning is demonstrated by a change in behaviour. At two a child may run into the street if the garden gate is left open. Within a few years he will usually have acquired the habit of stopping by the kerb to check for oncoming traffic. It is concluded that he has learned to cross the road safely. That learning has taken place is inferred because his behaviour has changed. Changed behaviour confirms learning. But what happened within the child to bring about the learning? From everyday observation we may reach a number of conclusions as to what may have gone on:

1. He may have learned from experience. Perhaps he stepped out and got hurt.
2. He may have learned because something frightened him. Perhaps he saw someone knocked down by a car.
3. He may have come to an understanding of danger and an acceptance of the need to avoid it, by being told stories or shown pictures.

These are reasonable explanations, as far as they go. They illustrate that there may be three ways to learn: through doing, feeling and thinking. In other words, the child's behaviour has changed because he now has a concept of danger related to motor cars and he has been motivated to avoid the danger. In this case the motivation may have come from fear, from experience or from an inculcated sense of responsibility. Another possible explanation would be that the avoidance of danger is an instinctual reaction. Human learning is complex. Learning theorists have provided a variety of explanations of how learning takes place and what motivates it.

The teaching-learning process

The process of teaching and learning for health is an interactive one: both learner and teacher have to be actively involved. Factors in the learner, the teacher and the teaching environment all create the teaching situation and influence the outcome of teaching and learning. The responsibility for what goes on in teaching and learning does not lie exclusively with any one of the partners in the process, nor can it either depend upon or be divorced from the environment in which it occurs. Figure 3.1 illustrates some of the interrelated factors in teaching and learning.

Health teaching should be designed to meet the needs of the learner and encourage accountability in both teacher and learner. A systematic but flexible approach is greatly preferable to episodic teaching. The use of a planned procedure helps both participants in the teaching–learning process to

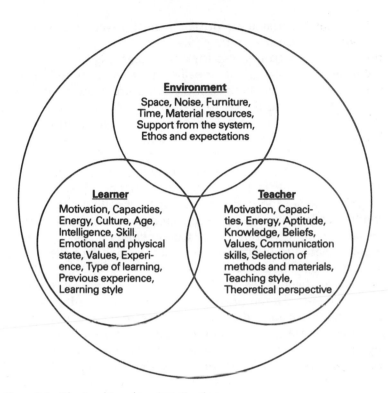

Figure 3.1 The teaching–learning situation

identify and focus on specific learning needs, to plan how to meet those needs, to put the plans into action and then to evaluate if learning occurred.

This approach approximates problem-solving mechanisms which people use, to greater or lesser extent, in their everyday lives. For instance, if several individuals discover that the bus route to the area where they live is about to be discontinued, they will usually explore the options open to them. Some might lobby for restitution of the service. Others might turn to using taxis. A few would weigh up the pros and cons of setting up a car pool or buying some type of vehicle such as a car, motorcycle, moped or bicycle, for transportation. The cost of each of these options would be considered in light of savings, income and maintenance costs. In the end, each individual would make a decision and put it into action. Those people who did not think carefully about the pros and cons might find out that their decision did not result in the best possible solution for them.

Using a planned process for health teaching means focussing upon what is needed. Ideally, the learner should participate at all stages to help identify what knowledge, attitudes and behaviours he needs to acquire in relation to his health status. A systematic approach to teaching and learning contributes to comprehensive assessment and renders accountability possible by promoting the prediction of success. It may also enhance efficiency in health care settings but this should not be the prime factor in utilising a planned process. Cost effectiveness as the main motivator for health teaching is in conflict with some values associated with concepts such as prevention and promotion. Cost-related goals are more usually related to institutions and professions, not client satisfaction or participation.

Problem-solving approaches to teaching and learning are characterised by attempts to ensure objectivity, rationality and applicability. Though these are desirable elements in any programme of care, they present certain dangers in health teaching, since they may encourage a mechanistic approach to assessing, planning and implementing teaching. Routine, even rigid, deployment of the health teaching process may be avoided by encouraging each patient or client to participate to the fullest degree possible in assessing learning needs and planning how the learning will take place. The unique nature of each individual and his idiosyncratic way of viewing his needs force the nurse to consider a world view which may differ radically from her own. Thus, each individual undergoing surgery, for instance, will have some common and some exclusive pre-operative learning needs. Health teaching as a planned process facilitates knowledgeable self-care, and promotes and accepts the responsibility of the individual for his own health decisions.

THEORETICAL CONSIDERATIONS

Learning theories

Most learning theories have been derived from experiments under laboratory-type conditions and as such they have to be applied with caution to everyday life. Nonetheless, learning theories help to interpret people's behaviour while learning and also can suggest solutions to some learning problems. Thus, the health teacher needs a basic understanding of two types of learning theory: associative and cognitive.

Associative learning theorists

These theorists claim that learning can be explained as a connection, made by the learner, between a stimulus and a response. The process by which such a connection is made has been labelled conditioning. Two types of conditioning have been distinguished: classical and operant (or instrumental). *Classical conditioning* was first described by Pavlov who noted that dogs salivated in response to the sight of food. He labelled this 'unconditioned response', because training was not needed to elicit it. He experimented by sounding a bell regularly before the dog's food was served and discovered that the dog could be trained to salivate upon hearing the bell, even when no food was given. This he labelled 'conditioned response'.

Operant conditioning

This is also an explanation of trained response but here the subject of the experiment 'operates' the environment in such a way as to receive a reward. Classic examples of 'operant' conditioning are the experiments carried out by a psychologist called Skinner who showed that pigeons exploring their boxes could be trained to operate a lever to deliver food. In this case the food was the reward for or 'reinforcer' of the learning. In a series of experiments, Skinner demonstrated that learning could be induced by administering carefully planned rewards which he called a schedule of reinforcements.

Cognitive learning theorists

These theorists on the other hand, stress the importance of ideas, perceptions and feelings in human learning. They offer explanations for more complex forms of learning, such as the learning involved when human beings solve problems or process information. Central to cognitive learning theories is the idea of *perception*, which is concerned with how human beings make sense of the world around them. Perception is the process which is said to be involved when individuals look at the same object but see it differently. In other words, the response to the stimulus (the object viewed) may differ because the individual's previous experience will influence how he perceives the object. Experiments have shown that both cultural expectations and past experience influence how individuals perceive things.

A group of well-known cognitive theorists are the *Gestalt* psychologists, who gave to the German word 'Gestalt', which means patterns, a new meaning in psychology when they used it to refer to 'wholes'. They suggested that breaking human behaviour down into small pieces was potentially distorting and that the true meaning of the behaviour was likely to be lost. Gestalt theorists recognised that the whole is sometimes greater than the sum of its parts and that people see and interpret things as a whole rather than by considering the bits and pieces that go to make up the picture. Gestalt psychologists were concerned to consider how the individual's perception of a situation would influence the way he responded to any given stimulus. They demonstrated the tendency for people to make sense of things by grouping items or seeing patterns.

An important idea from Gestalt psychology is that of *insight*. There are times when learning seems to happen all at once, the individual suddenly feels that he now understands. This has been described as the 'aha' reaction. Most people can recall such moments and sometimes it is even possible to observe them happening in other people. Having insight means suddenly seeing relationships which make the previously meaningless make sense. Gaining insight allows the individual to solve the immediate problem and apply what he has learned to similar situations in the future.

Types and levels of learning

Learning theorists have distinguished three types of learning: cognitive, affective and psychomotor:

— *Cognitive learning* refers to the process of thinking, of acquiring information and working with it.
— *Affective learning* is learning which incorporates the values, attitudes, beliefs and feelings which create idiosyncratic reactions. This kind of learning has important motivational influences.
— *Psychomotor skill learning* is the acquisition of a motor skill, such as self-injection or dressing change, through controlled neuromuscular movements. The skill is learned and perfected through practice.

It is generally acknowledged that there are different levels of learning, and that the process of learning may involve moving through a heirarchy; that is that the learner proceeds from the concrete to the abstract or from lower level skills to higher level skills. Gagné (1974), in his discussion of the acquisition of intellectual skills, lists eight categories of learning beginning with the simplest, the development of involuntary behaviour through classical conditioning. He proposes that an individual has to proceed through each category successfully before achieving the next level. The learner, after an initial period in which he merely recognises and responds to stimuli, will progress to more complex forms of learning such as verbal associations, differentiation of stimuli, concept formation and, finally, problem solving. One well-known classification of learning types and levels is Bloom's *Taxonomy* (Bloom, 1956; Krathwohl et al, 1964). Cognitive, affective and psychomotor learning levels proposed by Bloom and his colleagues are summarised in Table 3.1.

The existence of types and levels of learning has practical implications for the health teacher. It is important, in planning for teaching, to consider the level of learning which will be required. Does the pre-operative patient require facts only? Or facts plus understanding? Is it enough for the diabetic person to have a willingness to accept his diabetes? Or does he have to reach a point where beliefs about the value of self-care will lead to a life characterised by dietary and other disciplines? And if the latter is the case, what part can the nurse play as teacher and how much can be accomplished during a short hospital stay? Does the person with a stoma have to be able to innovate in managing appliances, or will it be

Table 3.1 Learning levels of the three types of learning (Bloom, 1956; Krathwohl et al, 1964)

Cognitive learning levels	Affective learning levels	Psychomotor learning levels
Knowledge—facts, concepts	Receiving—awareness	Perception—receiving sensory signals and translating
↓	↓	↓
Comprehension— understanding	Responding— willingness	Set—motivation
↓	↓	↓
Application—using knowledge	Valuing—commitment	Guided response— imitation, trial and error
↓	↓	↓
Analysis—seeing relationships of ideas	Organisation— discussion	Mechanism—learned response
↓	↓	↓
Synthesis—forming new patterns of thought, ideas	Characterisation— living the belief, value	Complex overt response—smooth response
↓		↓
Evaluation—critiquing value of ideas		Adaptation—altering response
		↓
		Origination— innovation with response

enough to follow mechanically the pattern set by the nursing staff in hospital? If he has to accomplish origination, by what stage in his post-operative progress will this be a reasonable expectation—immediately prior to discharge, at the first out-patients appointment or within one year of surgery?

If the learning process is hierarchical then conditions are imposed upon the teacher. It may be necessary to begin with the familiar and move to the unfamiliar. In helping a woman who is a new diabetic to understand the principle of asepsis in the injection technique, any experience she has of infant feeding could be utilised. It will also be important to consider individual differences. Each person acquires and uses knowledge in different ways. Personal styles of cognitive learning help to determine the health teaching approach which will achieve a positive learning outcome. Cognitive processes are involved in most adult psychomotor skill learning, for an understanding of the relevance of the skill has to be developed along with the acquisition of the skill movements. Reinforcement is thus a crucial tool in health teaching. Usually it will take the form of offering constructive feedback.

Motivation for learning

Motivation is a crucial factor influencing learning. Lefrancois (1982) asks 4 questions which are related to motivation and learning:

> What initiates action?
> What directs behaviour?
> Why is behaviour learned?
> Why does behaviour stop? (p. 301)

There are a number of possible explanations for what motivates human behaviour. The first is instinct. Earlier in the chapter it was suggested that the child who avoids danger by not running into the road may have acted instinctively. However, explaining complex human behaviours in this way raises questions. Lefrancois (1982) writes that the notion of instincts may be more appropriate to the behaviour of animals than humans, and states:

> Perhaps a mother, left to her own devices, would instinctively know how to deliver and care for her child. Perhaps not. In any event, experience, culture, and evolution have so modified our behaviour that the question of the existence of human instinct has become largely irrelevant. (p. 304)

Other theories have been devised to explain learning behaviour in terms of needs, and reactions to need. One, the *Need-drive theory* posits that when a need, be it physiological or psychological, occurs it creates a state of arousal or energy which works to satisfy the need. Frequently a motive is described in exactly those terms—as a force within a person which spurs him to achieve in some direction.

Maslow (1970) has proposed a *needs satisfaction theory* in which he feels that human beings strive to meet first their basic needs (physiological such as food, water and thermoregulation) before concerning themselves with higher level needs (safety, love and belongness and self esteem) culminating in self-actualisation. The higher level needs are achieved through a personal, therefore idiosyncratic, desire to develop and grow.

More recently, the *cognitive theory of motivation* has been proposed (Weiner, 1980). In this theory people are considered as active participants in creating their own motivation through desire to learn or in anticipation of learning. Thus, motivation is part of one's behaviour, not something which occurs in isolation. The Gestalt cognitive theorists discussed earlier presented motivation as a tension or force created by the difference between what the individual desires and achieves. McClelland and his colleagues (1953) developed an *achievement motivation theory* which is similar. Tensions set up within the individual force him to achieve to the degree which will ease the tension.

All of these theories have a common feature in that they assume some degree of *need* exists and that needs require a *response* of some sort to excite behaviour to ease the tension, and thus meet the need. *Arousal* is such a response and, in its simplest definition, refers to the degree of alertness within an individual. Visual and auditory senses are primary sources of arousal but Berlyne (1960) also found that certain properties of stimuli were important in arousal—novelty, meaningfulness, complexity and so on. Optimal arousal (or attention to the learning task) is conducive to learning. In people who are bored little learning will occur.

Anxiety is related to the level of arousal and at a high level may be detrimental to learning. The young woman who has a stoma created in surgery for cancer of the bowel may be so worried about the recurrence of cancer that her learning to care for her stoma may be inhibited.

The mechanism of arousal can be controlled to a certain degree by manipulating those variables which are external to the individual. For instance, if vision is an arousal source, the use of audio-visual aids will stimulate the learners as will a voice which avoids monotone qualities. The rule of thumb seems to be variety (Lefrancois, 1982) to evoke optimal levels of arousal for learning.

Two kinds of motivation are distinguished by psychologists: *intrinsic* motivation for those behaviours which continue without any observable rewards or reinforcement and *extrinsic* motivation which appears to depend on reinforcement. Extrinsic motivation persists only for a short period after reinforcement stops if the motivation has not become intrinsic. The need to encourage the development of intrinsic motivation in health teaching is clear. The distinction between the two types of motivation helps to explain the low rate of compliance with prescribed regimes. In hospital, reinforcement is provided by health care workers, the patient complies and rarely has the opportunity to create his own motivation by considering fully his health problem and its effects. With the withdrawal of reinforcement out of the hospital, the desired behaviour is likely to stop unless the patient has internalised the motivation to continue and therefore needs no external rewards.

The relationship of memory to learning

Early theories of learning were concerned with how change in knowledge and behaviour occurred. Theories about memory, on the other hand, deal with how knowledge is retained. In practice, memory and learning are very much interrelated. Any task of learning or memory depends upon the individual being able to perceive and transform knowledge from the environment (sometimes this is called encoding), attend to information presented and retrieve information already stored in the memory. The individual's ability to retain knowledge influences the extent of his comprehension and reasoning.

Memory is what helps individuals to maintain changed behaviour. In a person's memory is stored his attitudes, skills and his thinking strategies, all essential to learning.

In order to think, to reason, to learn, to remember or to recognise things as being meaningful or familiar it is necessary to be able to store large quantities of information. Storage of information is one function of memory, but storage alone is not enough. Consider a set of nursing journals. They represent a large store of information, but the information will be inaccessible unless indexed so that the various subjects dealt with may be identified and the information retrieved. Any store needs to be organised so that items held may be located and retrieved. Finding a book in a library or a drug in a medicine trolley, depends upon the existence of a reliable retrieval system. Similarly, human memory functions by having a system whereby information stored may be classified or categorised and subsequently retrieved. Such a system may be dependent upon the existence of different types of memory or levels of processing. There are three components of the memory system to consider:

1. *Immediate or sensory memory* is when there is immediate recognition of something but the memory is not stored for very long, only seconds. An example of this kind of memory would be to read through a list of items such as a shopping list, and then try to repeat it from memory a few seconds later.

2. *short-term memory* is longer than immediate memory but it still does not commit knowledge for later retrieval. Students who are busy writing notes in class exemplify this type of memory. They hold, in their minds, the material to be written. Once the writing is done, the memory fades. Remembering to put a date in one's diary is another instance. An active, ongoing process, short-term memory may be easily disturbed. If the person trying to remember to note a date in his diary is interrupted between agreeing to the date and writing it, that date may not appear in his diary without reinforcement.

3. *long-term memory* is more stable and not as easily disturbed. It is said to be constructive rather than reproductive which means that story-telling may be coloured or distorted. This accounts for the unreliability of eye witnesses to crimes.

Information may be passed between short and long-term memory, depending upon its salience to the individual. The exact interrelationship of parts of the memory system is not known but human memory is a multi-process operation, and whatever the storage system, memory seems to depend upon how information is processed for storage (Kintsch, 1977).

People process information for storage according to their prior knowledge. In memorising the nature of a collection of bottles containing liquid for drinking, the bottles might be categorised as:

3 green, 4 brown, 2 clear
or
2 large, 7 small
or
6 alcoholic beverages, 3 soft drinks
or
8 full, 1 empty

According to individual knowledge of contents, perception of the significance of certain characteristics of the bottles and knowledge of the purpose of the memory task.

Memory depends upon being able to store and retrieve information and is enhanced according to the individual's ability to categorise and organise material in a meaningful way. Processes by which memory may be enhanced are by combining items, by forming associations with items, or by rehearsing (repeating them over and over). The amount and timing of rehearsals can be all important in memory, as can knowledge of which items to rehearse. The practical applications of such features of memory are explored in Chapter 5 in relation to the presentation of factual information in health teaching.

People have their own individual approaches to processing information for remembering, and usually will remember best if allowed to utilise their own system (Mandler & Pearlstone, 1966). In general, however, events which are best remembered are either meaningful, organised, striking in a visual sense or overlearned. Various theories have been posited (Lefrancois, 1982) to account for forgetfulness and include the fading of memories not frequently recalled, the suppression of memories unpleasant to the individual and the inability of an individual to retrieve from his memory due to a poorly organised retrieval system. A further theory, *interference*, is a more recent explanation.

The theory of interference suggests that forgetting can occur in one of two ways: retroactively, or forgetting because something learned since has inhibited the memory; and proactively, or forgetting because previous learning has inhibited the memory. Simply put, sometimes prior learning adversely affects memory, other times it is subsequent learning which causes forgetting.

The adult as learner

Adults learn differently from children for a number of reasons which encompass aspects of the physical as well as the psychological state.

Physical effects of ageing

Although cognitive functioning does not necessarily decline with age there are ageing effects which may in turn affect learning. Vision begins to deteriorate early in life, but is most noticeable after the age of forty. The normal eye at the age of twenty admits twice the amount of light as does the pupil in a 50 year old. Other vision deficits include decreased recovery from glare effects, slower accommodation to darkness and a gradual decrease in colour sensitivity. These changes may be critical, as much of what an individual learns is by sight. Hearing is affected by age, with a loss of auditory acuity for high-pitched sounds. The other senses of taste, touch and smell may decrease only gradually.

With age, psychomotor skill learning slows due to changes in the neuromuscular system. Reaction times increase and teachers find that older learners take longer to follow directions or to respond to questions. Accuracy does not diminish if the older individual is left to work at his own pace.

Short-term memory is also affected by ageing. The process is more prone to disruption by intervening activity. Again, by allowing the individual to pace himself, the results can equal the performance of younger learners. Table 3.2 summarises the physical changes occurring with ageing and suggests how to compensate for them in health teaching situations.

Age and psychological manifestations

Jennifer Rogers (1977) has noted a number of reactions which

Table 3.2 Summary of physical effects of ageing and compensatory actions

Physical effects of ageing	Compensatory actions

1. Vision—pupillary size ↓
    —colour sensitivity ↓
    —recovery from glare ↓
	1. —if using printed material, print must be readable
	—increase no-glare lighting
	—use strong colours in audiovisual aids (green, red, black)

2. Hearing— ↓ high pitched sounds	2. —speak distinctly, not shrilly —control environmental distractions
3. Psychomotor—reaction time ↑	3. —allow self-paced activity
4. Memory—short term ↓	4. —keep directions to a minimum, reinforce oral instruction with written material —develop learning materials in manageable amounts

may be seen in the adult learner. First, the older learner may be anxious about appearing foolish if concepts or skills are not grasped quickly. Such risk-taking may not be seen as worthwhile since the adult's status and self-esteem may be threatened.

The question of risk to status and self-esteem has particular relevance in health teaching, since teaching so often takes place in situations, like a hospital, a surgery or clinic in which people feel at a disadvantage or in circumstances, such as illness, which reduce confidence. Additionally, the person's usual claims to status such as occupation and socio-economic position may be temporarily threatened, or at the very least not immediately obvious. Such considerations may all lead to lack of self-confidence in the learner, and thus present barriers to learning.

Another reaction contributing adversely to the learning process may be the individual's view of ageing. He may believe that 'you can't teach an old dog new tricks.' Also, the memories of past learning experiences may colour the learner's motivation to participate. If learning has presented problems in the past there may be expectation of a further negative experience.

A final consideration in adult learning is social background. Social distance between teacher and learner may be more important in adults than in children. Additionally, the adult will have formed attitudes to his control over his destiny, and over illness in particular, to aspects of health and disease and to learning itself, all of which will influence his willingness and ability to learn.

It is important to remember that the adult learner may not be willing to learn about his health and that he may not find it easy to learn. Respect for and acceptance of the adult learner will go a long way to overcoming some of his personal and emotional reactions to learning. It is vitally important to acknowledge and use the experience of adult learners and to build upon existing knowledge and experience.

SOME THINGS TO REMEMBER ABOUT LEARNING

1. Learning may be conscious or unconscious

There is such a thing as latent learning. Some people can name all the shops in their local high street, though they have not ever consciously set themselves the task of learning what is there; their knowledge has been acquired subconsciously, by latent learning. Some people have a greater capacity for latent learning than others, but everyone does some subconscious learning by picking up cues from the environment. Patients and clients pick up cues from the hospital or clinic environment and from health professionals. Some of them will be more aware of cues than others, but the cues do matter: they contribute to subconscious learning.

If there is subconscious learning then it follows that there may be subconscious teaching. Some cues people pick up from health professionals are transmitted intentionally. Other cues may be ones the health professionals would want to disown.

2. Learning occurs when the individual is able to learn

Clearly, a cluster of interrelated factors such as age, sex, social class and educational level may be expected to influence the individual's learning capabilities. Factors of particular relevance to the nurse as health teacher, however, are:

The developmental stage of the learner

It will be obvious that teaching a young child will require a very different process to teaching an adult. But exactly how should such differences be incorporated in planned health teaching? The work of Friedland (1976), an American nurse, is a useful illustration of how nurses may apply an understanding of human learning to nursing care. Friedland observed the learning process of an 11-year-old boy newly diagnosed as having diabetes mellitus. She noticed two important things. Firstly, he had to concentrate very hard in the early stages of learning to inject himself with insulin and to test his urine for sugar. She noticed that if any explanations were given whilst he was handling equipment he had to stop what he was doing to listen: he simply could not do two things at once. That is well worth remembering. Nurses are busy people, who often attempt two jobs at once. It is quite tempting to save time by giving people explanations whilst they are practising. Friedland's observations suggest that this is not always a good idea and that it may be important for the nurse to keep quiet while someone practises.

The second thing Friedland noted was that it was fully four days before the boy could manage abstract ideas. Again, this is important. Asepsis is a difficult concept to grasp and some people may need a sequence of lessons. Learning is a process of steps and stages, which the nurse should gear to the developmental stage of the individual.

The language used

No one will have the ability to understand health teaching if the language used is inappropriate. Clearly, language ability relates to age, socio-economic and cultural factors, but the person's ability to understand will also be governed by the nurse's willingness to use language he can understand. Means of avoiding jargon and using and explaining technical terms are discussed in detail in Chapter 5.

Pain and denial

It is important to remember that nurses often teach in very difficult circumstances. Whenever possible, teaching should be postponed when someone is in pain. The psychological mechanism of denial may be more difficult to deal with since it is often quite long-standing, but it is important to realise that it may exist and that it will be necessary to set realistic objectives which take sensible account of what can be expected of learners and nurses alike.

3. Learning occurs when the individual is willing to learn

The key to learning is motivation, and the essence of teaching is to motivate the learner. In health teaching, factors to consider are:

The level of anxiety

This can assist or hinder learning: moderate anxiety may help people to learn about their health, by motivating them to avoid disease or disability. The role of fear-arousing messages in motivating people to health actions is further discussed in Chapter 4. However, high anxiety may cause people to resist a message or simply fail to hear it. In general terms, the role of the nurse in health teaching will usually be to allay high levels of anxiety.

Learner satisfaction

This is motivating. The way to achieve this is to set realistic goals. When goals are too easy, people do not try to learn; goals outwith their grasp cause people to give up without trying.

Having meaningful material aids learning

People learn more quickly when the material presented makes sense to them.

4. Active use of material aids learning

Anyone who has prepared for an examination knows that active use of information helps aid understanding and memory. Discussing issues with a friend, drawing diagrams or making word pictures all help to grasp hold of the material to be reproduced on the day of examination. Active learning is equally important in health teaching. With a wide range of learners, nurses have to be imaginative as health teachers to involve people in active learning. An example of work done by Canadian nurses with diabetic children illustrates the scope for active involvement. Leahy et al (1975) decided that since children learn so readily through play, diabetic education might be effective if devised as games. They produced a learning package for 6–12 year olds which had a separate format for different age groups in that range, planning for five main teaching areas: the pathophysiology of diabetes, the administration and storage of insulin, urine testing, the relationship of food, exercise and insulin to blood glucose and insulin reaction and ketoacidosis. It was a lot to tackle, but there is a great deal to teach in diabetic education. Lessons were spaced over time and also involved the children's parents. Amongst the materials produced were: a flannelgraph about the body, which the children played with as they learned some simple anatomy; a doll, syringe and needles with which the children played out feelings of being attacked when injected by their parents; and, food models and scales which allowed the children and their parents to consider food values as they played together.

5. Learning is emotional as well as intellectual

In the example quoted above (Leahy et al, 1975), the plans for active learning included affective learning because it is such an important aspect of learning in relation to diabetes mellitus. In health teaching generally, it is necessary to remember that there are routes to learning through feeling as well as thinking and experience and that all three may have to be considered. Also, it is essential to remember that health teaching will usually involve the feelings and beliefs of both learner and nurse.

6. Learning is sometimes painful

It can be difficult to learn new material. Health learning may be especially difficult, since cherished beliefs are sometimes challenged.

7. Learning arises out of experience

It is important to remember that there are some things people can only learn by being given the experience of doing them for themselves. This presents nurses with some difficulties in practice. For instance, learning to accept responsibility for drugs will depend upon being given responsibility for handling drugs. It is not enough to exhort the individual to be responsible when he gets home: he may need to be given the chance to manage his regimen whilst in hospital. Letting the individual assume responsibility may have logistical as well as legal implications. For instance, stoma management self-care by the individual may in fact consume much more professional time than if the nurse were to carry out the procedure.

SOME THINGS TO REMEMBER ABOUT TEACHING

1. Know the learner's capacities

Before anyone can be taught anything, their capacities for learning have to be assessed. Intelligence level, age and learning experience have to be noted. Cultural, ethnic and religious differences may affect learning. What is the learner's state? The person who is mentally handicapped may never understand the use of digitalis for a cardiac condition. This seems an obvious consideration but it may prove difficult to assess. The young man who is obese knows that his level of health is negatively affected by the excess weight, but his eating patterns will not change because eating provides one of the few pleasures in his life. His motivation is not conducive to change. Assessment of the learner is further discussed in Chapter 6.

2. Motivate the learner

Motivation is the key to learning. The keen learner attends to what is to be learned. The motives may be intrinsic to the person or applied externally, but the learner who is intrinsically motivated learns more readily and remembers the learning over a longer period of time.

3. Provide for learner activity

When the learner is actively engaged in his own learning it becomes more meaningful. Demonstrating how to inject insulin to a group of diabetic patients and then expecting them to proceed with injecting themselves is unreasonable. They need to handle the equipment in order to be able to gain confidence. By practising injection, say of an orange, they learn the feel of the syringe, they learn how to balance it and how to angle it for a subcutaneous injection. The procedure means something to their senses as well as their minds.

4. Reinforce progress

The knowledge of success is motivating. Learning can be a lonely business. The middle-aged woman on a diet may feel encouraged if weight loss is recorded on her bathroom scales. She will often feel even greater reward if others note and applaud her progress and so a health teaching programme might include regular 'check-ins' with others present.

5. Give feedback

While the previous principle related to success, it should be noted that one may learn from one's mistakes. Feedback should be related to the event and should be given in a helpful manner. Feedback guides the learner to know the limits of his learning and to become more proficient, skilled or sensitive, depending on the task at hand. Telling someone that what he is doing is 'wrong' may obstruct learning. Suggesting that there 'may be another way of trying that' helps the learner to compare different approaches and to decide which is more effective.

6. Plan the teaching

A teacher's familiarity with the material evokes a response of respect. The nurse is seen as the expert and if she is undertaking to teach about a topic she must have a firm knowledge base. Nowadays, nurses have to teach people who may be as well informed about their illness as are the health professionals who care for them. Some people study their particular health problem in great detail and are familiar with the most recent advances and the different causation theories proposed. This knowledge can be profitably shared by the patient and, in fact, may provide the motivating force for interaction to learn other things.

7. Check the teaching image

A teacher must be consistent, trustworthy and sincere. Respect for the learner must be evident. Nurses who help patients to control their weight are not effective models if they themselves are overweight. The nurse's enthusiasm for an activity can be catching. A group of adolescents who talk to a health visitor about jogging and discover that she jogs daily and has anecdotes about her experiences while jogging may see it as an activity they would like to try.

8. Practise recognising the 'teachable moment'

The 'teachable moment' refers to the instance when insight is about to occur. It is the time to stay with the learner so that she is able to grasp the meaning of something. To leave at that crucial time may mean several sessions to return to the same point of learning.

9. Facilitate discovery learning

In discovery learning, the learners see relationships in the material for themselves. To take the example of learning how to inject oneself, the nurse could present the learner with an instruction sheet and the materials and leave her to figure out how to open the disposable syringe package and how to fit the needle to the syringe. Then the learner could demonstrate and explain how she managed. This approach involves the learner and may be more meaningful for some learners.

10. Encourage self-evaluation

Through self-evaluation the learner demonstrates acceptance of the responsibility for learning. The diabetic patient who keeps up with the latest news through the newsletter of the

British Diabetic Association demonstrates this principle. Intrinsic motivation replaces extrinsic motivation. This necessitates the professionals being prepared to acknowledge to the individual at the outset that one day he may know as much as they do about the health problem, even to accept that he may know more, since he lives with it.

11. Be realistic

A chapter such as this one usually builds an idealised picture, conveying the impression that teaching and learning may be clearly defined and closely controlled. The truth of the matter is that there are good days and bad days. Sometimes people do not want to learn. The state of the learner and the teacher can affect learning. Mistakes will be made. The essence of good teaching is to examine what went well and what went badly and to use that knowledge for the future.

THE NURSE AS HEALTH TEACHER

Learning can be a most challenging, satisfying and sometimes painful experience. The individual who becomes personally involved in his own health and motivated to act responsibly and creatively, illustrates the ultimate aim of health teachers.

It has been indicated that the learning and teaching process is an interactive one, a mutual process. To achieve this sense of mutuality, a commitment is required from both participants and should include personal involvement with ideas, the programme and each other, as well as others. As teacher the nurse must be able to share her true self, to demonstrate an adequate personality and to acquire the self-discipline she will ask of her learners. What is called for is 'self-knowledge'. The health teacher frequently interacts with learners who may be older and better educated. This situation can cause heightened anxiety in the teacher. Recognition of personal limitations and coming to terms with them is a necessary step.

The health teacher is responsible for setting the atmosphere for learning. The ultimate goal is not only for the learner to develop as a knowledgeable being but also as a person. The qualities of the teacher affect the learning situation: being sincere, genuine, a person with vitality, convictions and feelings; caring for the learner, prizing him, accepting him as a unique individual and being empathetic.

The health teacher uses encounters to listen and to communicate, not to self-articulate. She must be reliable, consistent and have a strong self-concept which can admit to error. She is committed to health and to teaching as a way to enhance life. She is flexible and able to accept new ideas, changes and challenges from the learners and from contemporaries. These are demanding requirements, but no more so than other qualities of the professional nurse.

Effective health teaching occurs in an environment which is supportive, non-judgemental and unhurried and in which the learners are encouraged and facilitated to develop in ways which are most meaningful to them.

The learner who has experienced the best of what health teaching can do leaves the learning situation and:

1. values his own worth, his feelings and reactions;
2. has faith in his own ability to achieve;
3. gains insight into his own motivation and behaviour;
4. feels responsible for himself and others;
5. has experienced freedom though self-direction in learning, and
6. feels satisfied with the learning.

REFERENCES

Bloom B S (ed) 1956 Taxonomy of educational objectives, handbook 1: cognitive domain. David McKay Company, New York
Berlyne D E 1960 Conflict, arousal and curiosity. McGraw-Hill, New York
Friedland G M 1976 Learning behaviour of a pre-adolescent with diabetes. American Journal of Nursing 76(1): 59–61
Gagné R M 1974 Essentials of learning for instruction. Dryden Press, Hinsdale, Illinois
Krathwohl D K, Bloom B S, Masia B B 1964 Taxonomy of educational objectives, handbook 11: affective domain. David McKay Company, New York
Kintsch W 1977 Memory and cognition. John Wiley and Sons, New York
Leahy M D, Logan S A, McArthur R G 1975 Paediatric diabetes: a new teaching approach. Canadian Nurse 71(10): 18–20
Lefrancois G R 1982 Psychology for teaching. 4th edn. Wadsworth Publishing Company, Belmont, California
Mandler G, Pearlstone Z 1966 Free and constrained concept learning and subsequent recall. Journal of Verbal Learning and Verbal Behaviour 5: 126–131

Maslow A H 1970 Motivation and personality, 2nd edn. Harper and Row, New York
McClelland D C, Atkinson J W, Clark R A, Lowell E L 1953 The achievement motive. Appleton-Century-Crofts, New York
Rogers J 1977 Adults learning, 2nd edn. The Open University Press, Milton Keynes
Turner J S, Helms D B 1979 Contemporary adulthood. W B Saunders, London
Weiner B 1980 Human motivation. Holt, Rinehart & Winston, New York

FURTHER READING

Hill W F 1963 Learning. University Paperbacks, Methuen, London
Howe M J A 1980 The psychology of human learning. Harper & Row, New York
Norman D A 1976 Memory and attention: an introduction to human information processing. John Wiley & Sons, New York

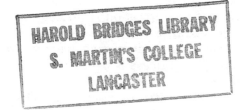

4

Therapeutic and persuasive communication

OBJECTIVES

Study of this chapter will enable you to:

1. Describe what is meant by therapeutic communication.
2. Identify techniques of therapeutic communication.
3. Identify factors which influence the process of communication.
4. Discuss factors which enhance the success of persuasive communication.

The word communication connotes sharing. To communicate means to represent a message and to send it to another person through a medium such as sight, smell, taste, touch or hearing. The process is dynamic and it occurs constantly, whether or not we are aware of it. Communication may be oral or written, verbal or nonverbal. All interaction involves communication. Talking with a friend, stopping in the street to greet a neighbour, visiting the doctor, sharing grief at the death of a favourite pet, arguing with a teacher about a maths problem, widening eyes in disbelief and shrugging one's shoulders in disgust all involve communication. What was said? How was it said? What was meant? What was implied without words? How was the message received by the person to whom it was directed? Such questions illustrate that communication is not mere 'talking', but a complex process which is part of our daily lives.

Communication is a two way process, involving passing messages to and fro, between a sender and a receiver. Figure 4.1 illustrates a simple model of communication.

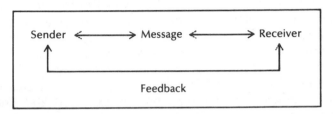

Figure 4.1 A communication model

Communication plays an important role in nursing. Nurses have to be skilled communicators in order to identify patient or client needs, assist in the expression of needs, aid the understanding of preventive activity, treatment or care, and facilitate the acquisition of self-care skills. To be effective communicators nurses have to be skilled receivers as well as senders of messages.

In health teaching, communication is a planned process which is effective when the client attains certain goals. Health teaching is integral to the normal process of therapeutic communication between nurse and patient.

THERAPEUTIC COMMUNICATION

Therapeutic communication in nursing has been described (Gazda et al, 1975) as a three phase cycle of helping, involving facilitation, transition and action phases. The essential features of the *facilitation phase* are talking and listening in a manner which is empathetic, warm, non-directive and non-judgemental. It is necessary to respect the individual and to accept his interpretation of events. Such a situation reduces threat and the client is more able to speak freely, release emotions and explore the problem. The basis of the therapeutic relationship is being laid. The *transition phase* requires more intervention. When the patient has reached a saturation point and cannot take self-exploration and understanding any further without help, the nurse can ask specific relevant questions. At this point the nurse needs to demonstrate interest and 'genuineness', and may use self-disclosure if such a tactic is appropriate. Saying 'I've been there too' can be helpful but only if the patient remains the focus. In the transition phase the patient's problem is defined. In the *action phase* problem solving begins. The nurse helps the patient to plan strategies. Confrontation about discrepancies in what the patient says and does may be needed. The patient who says 'I am overweight and will now diet' but who eats chocolates frequently, may be confronted providing he has explored and understands his motivations for action.

In all helping relationships termination must occur. Throughout the 'process of helping', both participants are learning about one another, the situation and the problem. A relationship is formed and must be ended when the patient no longer requires the help of the nurse.

It is all too easy to represent therapeutic communication as a straightforward sequential process and easily acquired skill. In fact, for most nurses, neophyte and experienced, it means learning a new skill and trying to break old habits. In the first trial of a new skill such as bathing a patient or changing a dressing, the nurse may find that her movements are awkward. She has to stop and think about principles and procedure and the whole process moves rather slowly. Eventually, with practice, the nurse becomes adept. The process of communicating therapeutically is attained in the same way. Awkwardness and artificiality accompany the first few efforts. With practice and regular review the skill becomes smoother, easier and more effective.

THE COMMUNICATION PROCESS

Analysis of what happens in given communications can provide clues to understanding the process of communication. Consider, for instance, the following except from a conversation between a staff nurse from a general surgical ward and a pre-operative patient:

Nurse (on entering hospital room at 0930 hours): 'Good morning, Mr Keighley. I've come to talk with you about your operation.'

Mr Keighley (looking worried): 'Is there anything wrong? I mean, is everything still on for tomorrow?'

Nurse (brightly): 'Oh, yes, the operation is still scheduled for tomorrow. I've come to explain some of the procedures which will occur before the operation and to answer any questions you might have.'

Mr Keighley: 'Oh, that's all right, then.'

Elements of communication

In the above exchange there are six identifiable elements:

1. *The motivating reason* for the exchange or the idea behind it. The nurse approached Mr Keighley for pre-operative preparation and her reason was the need to communicate about what to expect before and after surgery.

2. *The sender,* or the person initiating the conversation, in this case the nurse. How the nurse converses will be affected by her level of skill in communicating, her attitude towards the situation (does she feel Mr Keighley has no right to be worried as his surgeon has a very good reputation?), her level of knowledge about the surgical procedure (will it be painful, how long does it take to come out of the anaesthetic, what does the surgeon do?) and her sociocultural background which includes her professional preparation.

3. *The message* is the actual expression relayed to the other person. How it is conveyed is important. Does it make sense or is it a jumble of words? Has there been a decision about the content? Will there be a reference to 'procedures before operation' or 'pre-operative information' or 'reducing surgical risks'? The content of the message must be closely considered or the patient will be left in confusion.

4. *The channel* refers to the way the message is sent. In the example, the nurse appeared before Mr Keighley and spoke to him, thereby stimulating the senses of sight and hearing. Other senses such as touch, taste and smell can be used in appropriate circumstances. An American nurse, Dolores Kreiger, has researched into the use of touch in caring for

patients. This 'laying on of hands' constitutes a special kind of 'listening' (Kreiger et al, 1979; Mason & Pratt, 1980).

5. *The receiver* is the person to whom the message is directed. The message has to be received and understood. If Mr Keighley had not seen or heard the nurse entering the room, he would not have recognised the fact that she was addressing him. The receiver's communication skills, knowledge level, attitudes and sociocultural background all influence how he participates.

6. *Feedback* is the final stage in which Mr Keighley responded to the nurse to let her know he understood that she was speaking to him on a particular topic, his scheduled surgery.

Figure 4.2 depicts a model of the communication process. The arrows in the figure circumscribe a full circle to indicate that the receiver heard the message. The feedback to the sender might be 'I understand' or 'I don't understand' or 'Can you repeat that?' In this way the process has been completed. If the receiver responded (gave feedback) and added something which sent a message which asked for a response, then the original sender becomes a receiver. The process is dynamic and messages can be sent in both directions, alternately or at the same time. Figure 4.3 illustrates such a situation.

The dynamic of communication

While the spoken word is sometimes considered to be the major manner of communicating, other aspects may affect the process. To distinguish these aspects, the term *verbal* refers to the words spoken, *paraverbal* describes how those words are said and *nonverbal* indicates the body language employed while communicating. Paraverbal and nonverbal modes may be just as important as verbal communication.

As an example of paraverbal communication, consider a patient saying to a nurse: 'I can't do what you are asking. It's impossible.' This sentence could be interpreted differently if the patient said it (1) calmly (2) loudly (3) screaming and emphasising the 'you' in the sentence. The way the voice is used: the volume, the tone, the tempo, the emphasis—all these aspects help to convey what the patient means. Authors of fiction have to be careful about inserting the paraverbal aspect

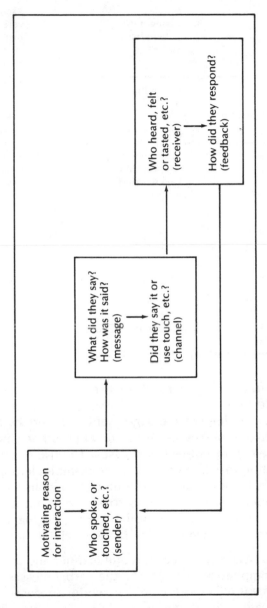

Figure 4.2 Model illustrating the process of communication

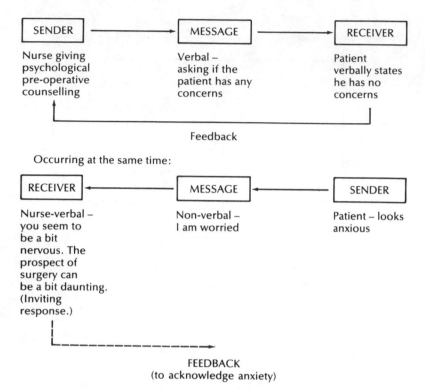

Figure 4.3   Example of messages being sent simultaneously

of their characters' speech, otherwise the conversations in books would be flat.

Body language implies messages sent to others by the way a person stands, makes gestures, touches others, positions himself in relation to others or dresses. The use of nonverbal communication may be conscious, for example, letting someone know that you are angry with him; or unconscious, as in the case where a person is feeling low in spirit but is unaware that people around him have noticed. Body language is used for many reasons (Argyle, 1975; Hargie et al, 1981):

1. It communicates in a clear forceful manner and may complement, emphasise or reinforce the verbal message.
2. Sometimes it tells more than the sender suspects.
3. It can create a visual impression in cases where words are not readily descriptive; for example, with shapes.

4. It is a convenient way of communicating and provides a choice of using two channels—the verbal and the nonverbal.

Analysis of communication, then, includes the verbal, the paraverbal, and the nonverbal.

TECHNIQUES OF THERAPEUTIC COMMUNICATION

While a number of techniques are utilised in therapeutic communication and are referred to in this chapter, three techniques are more fully described here because they constitute essential communication devices. These are: questioning, use of silence and interviewing.

Questioning

Questioning is a skill which helps:

1. to gain information about the patient's level of knowledge, his attitudes, opinions and feelings
2. to focus on particular subject matter
3. to express an interest or indicate attention
4. to involve the other person
5. to encourage self-exploration
6. to hold attention
7. to validate facts and observations
8. to clarify meanings.

The type of question may influence its effects. An *open-ended question* allows someone to describe or to elaborate on a topic. The nurse can ask: 'How did you feel when the doctor said you would need major surgery?' The *closed or direct question* asks for specific information and focusses the interview. A patient who has come into Accident and Emergency with severe chest pain will be asked 'Where is the pain? Does it radiate?' *Leading questions* do what they describe, they 'lead' the respondent to give the 'correct' response which the questioner expects when asking: 'You have been careful of your diet, haven't you?' This type of question is not helpful but is, unfortunately, common.

Silence

The use of silence as a mechanism for communication can be skilful. Silences in conversation may be uncomfortable but in therapeutic communication they serve a useful purpose as they can give the patient time to think, to remember, or to formulate a response. Sometimes silence is a natural pause in the flow of the talking; at other times, it creates a feeling of embarrassment. During silence the nurse can observe the patient's nonverbal behaviour and maintain an attitude which clearly invites the other person to go on talking. It can be difficult to judge when silence would be both comfortable and appropriate but it is important not to assume that every pause should be filled with talk!

Interviewing

Through the use of interviewing, therapeutic caring can be facilitated and improved. The interview is a process in which understanding of a situation is gained through the collection of information from the individual who is then helped to make decisions about his health status. Garrett (1972) has noted:

> Warm human interest does sometimes vanish from interviewing, and when that happens it becomes a monotonous, mechanical sort of thing that is relatively valueless. But the cause of this kind of interviewing, when it occurs, is not knowledge of the rich interplay of one human mind with another, but the ignorance that regards interviewing as a routine affair of asking set questions and recording answers. (p. 5)

Thus, the interview should be conducted skilfully with an atmosphere of support in which rapport between the nurse and patient facilitates self-exploration. The amount of self-exploration depends on the purpose of the interview. Three types of interviewing illustrate different purposes.

1. The structured interview

This is conducted to obtain specific information and it is seen as appropriate in cases of crisis. The nurse controls the pace of the interview. This type of interview has a particular place in crisis situations and with people who are acutely ill, where a leisurely talk will not provide sufficiently quickly essential details about the person. The structured interview may also be the first of a series of interviews, some of which may be semistructured or unstructured. The nurse may decide to begin in a structured manner to gain specific information which will be needed to make initial care plans. In a structured interview all questions are decided in advance, in accordance with the specific information to be gained.

2. The semistructured interview

This can be used not only to gain specific information but also to explore feelings or to promote patient participation. For instance, when caring for antenatal patients the nurse will want to know how the pregnancy is progressing and will collect information on weight, urine testing and physical changes. However, the feelings of the expectant woman will be important also. Does she want this baby? Is she having any fears about the labour and delivery period? Concerns such as these can be probed by encouraging the patient to talk. In such an interview only some of the questions are decided in advance.

3. The unstructured interview

This can be valuable in exploring feelings. The health visitor who would like to help high school students to explore how they see health in relation to themselves can use an unstructured format. She will not want to force her values and attitudes on the students, she will want them to question themselves about their own level of health, so that questions are not determined in advance, but allowed to arise.

As a communication tool, the interview should reflect the pattern of facilitation, transition and action described for therapeutic communication.

1. Set the stage. The interview begins by attending to the setting factors (the furniture, the lighting), by putting the patient at ease and offering openings to begin the exchange. The nurse facilitates the process by being empathetic, warm, encouraging and respectful.

2. *Build on the work started.* Questioning can help the patient to further explore the problem, to decide what the problem is, and to make decisions about acting on it.

3. *Close the interview.* Nursing interviews frequently have time limits. Keeping this in mind is important as an abrupt departure from the patient may be unsettling and can destroy the trust which has been built up. There should be time to review what has been discussed, to summarise the state of affairs, to note what progress has been made, and to focus on finishing. Asking the patient, 'Is there anything else you'd like to say today?' allows him the choice of terminating and tells him that the exchange will continue when next arranged.

At the end of an interview its effectiveness should be evaluated. Did helpful information emerge? Who did most of the talking? Did the nurse use herself effectively as a therapeutic agent? What was the patient's behaviour? Was the setting conducive? Was the problem situation identified by the patient? What decisions were made? Evaluation of the 'professional conversation' (Garrett, 1972) occurring between the nurse and the patient reveals whether or not caring was facilitated and improved.

PERSUASIVE COMMUNICATION

Sooner or later every nurse involved in health teaching will face the challenge of deciding whether or not it is right to persuade others to change behaviour, and how to achieve persuasion if this seems necessary or desirable.

In today's society everyone has experience of persuasion, either as persuader or as recipient of a would-be persuasive message. So everyone has ideas about what will persuade: choose arguments to fit the audience; get the language or even the pronunciation right; use vivid descriptions and good anecdotes; vary the tone of voice and manipulate body language; exploit rhyme and rhythm, figures of speech, cliche and paradox; demonstrate authority; amuse; charm; appeal to reason or to the emotions. These are all very familiar tricks in daily use in attempts at political persuasion and in any society subjected to the free forces of advertising. Visual impact is another important aspect of persuasion: consider the symbolism of the cross or the swastica. Today, television is the most obvious exploiter of visual impact, but ancillary media such as badges, beer mats, pens, key-rings and T-shirts are increasingly used to sell a product or an image. The emotive power of music is also exploited.

Most people can recall at least one advertising jingle, even if they have never bought the product. Other techniques widely believed to be successful in persuasion are repetition, enthusiasm, intimidation and audience participation.

In health education, persuasive techniques are directed at bringing about changes in attitudes or behaviour. Broadly, there are three sets of assumptions made about how this may be done. These are reflected in three main approaches to persuasion among health educators. Table 4.1 lists these approaches, all of which have two things in common. First, there is the assumption that beliefs, attitudes and behaviour are central concerns in persuading people to change actions related to health. Second, it is implied that there is some link between belief, attitude and behaviour.

Table 4.1 Three main approaches to persuasion among health educators

1. Education	: E X P L O R E attitudes and behaviour R E W A R D change
2. Propaganda	: M A N I P U L A T E attitudes and behaviour
3. Community development	: A S S I S T discovery of attitudes and behaviour A C C E P T the initiation or rejection of change

It is beyond the scope of this text to deal with problems of defining terms such as belief and attitude, but in considering persuasion it is useful for practical purposes to distinguish between opinions, attitudes and beliefs. One way to do this is to consider the extent to which they are involved with the personality of the individual. It is generally accepted that beliefs are central to the individual's personality structure, attitudes are less firmly attached, and opinions only peripherally attached. The belief system provides a framework for all that the person thinks and does, and governs how the individual will receive messages by a process which has been labelled 'selective perception'. The difference between an attitude and a belief is that an attitude always has an object and a direction. Attitudes may be described as positive or negative. Beliefs, on the other hand, are neutral.

These differences in the nature of opinions, attitudes and beliefs have implications for persuasion research. Different techniques may be needed to measure each. For instance, direct questioning will reveal opinions and even certain attitudes; however, the attitudes and beliefs most likely to be of interest to the health educator, such as beliefs about sexual practice or attitudes to abortion, are likely to be elicited only by more indirect, in-depth techniques. There are also important differences in relation to persuasive communication. Clearly, it is more likely that opinions will be changed more readily than attitudes and beliefs which have a more central position in the personality structure.

The link between beliefs, attitudes and behaviour

One of the questions which has challenged researchers looking at persuasive communication is how beliefs, attitudes and behaviour are linked. Traditional health education approaches have assumed that knowledge preceded attitudes, which would both predict and precede behaviour. The Knowledge–Attitude–Practice (KAP) model of health education is an example of this assumption. Figure 4.4 illustrates the KAP model. The model suggests that the right information will influence attitudes and thus change behaviour. Now it is accepted that this approach is naive and the relationship between knowledge, attitudes and behaviour is acknowledged as being more complex. Some types of information change some people's attitudes some of the time, but the knowledge–attitude–behaviour link is neither consistent nor unidirectional. Changing attitudes does not seem to guarantee a change in

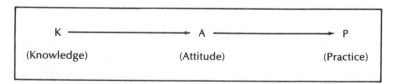

Figure 4.4 The KAP model for health education

behaviour. Additionally, it is known that changes in behaviour may bring about changes in attitude.

Fishbein & Ajzen (1981) have proposed that clusters of beliefs influence the formation of specific attitudes which in turn determine an individual's intention to act. Figure 4.5 illustrates this idea. Everyday experience, however, indicates that people do not always behave as they intend. The gap between intention and behaviour remains the major challenge to health educators. Somewhere in that gap there is an as yet unexplained interaction of strength of motivation versus the context in which health-related actions take place (Fig. 4.6).

For a time, the idea of any attitude–behaviour link was seriously questioned by researchers. This was because some

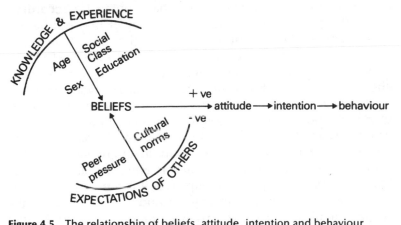

Figure 4.5 The relationship of beliefs, attitude, intention and behaviour

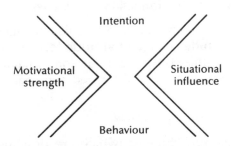

Figure 4.6 The intention–behaviour gap

research studies appeared to demonstrate that attitudes were not reliable predictors of behaviour. The first, and most famous of these, was published by La Piere (1934). He recorded that when a Chinese couple, accompanied by a Caucasian, toured restaurants and hotels in the United States of America they were refused admission at only one of 251 establishments. This was despite the fact that 92% of the owners said in response to a postal survey that they would not admit Chinese. Thus, doubt was cast on the assumed link between attitude and behaviour. However, recent reviews of the research (Ajzen & Fishbein, 1977; Petty et al, 1981) reveal that shortcomings in research design and methodology may account for the inconsistencies between attitude and behaviour which have been recorded. Firstly, attitudes are very difficult to measure and some researchers have opted for recording a verbal report of the attitude, which may or may not be the same thing as the attitude itself. Also, other aspects of some of the studies can be questioned. For instance, in the La Piere case, it is possible that managers handled the written query about reservations but other staff members dealt with the face-to-face encounters. Clearly, if different people were sampled there would be no reason to expect an attitude–behaviour link. Petty et al (1981) concludes that it can be assumed that there is, after all, a link between attitude and behaviour. What cannot be assumed is that that link is either linear or simple. Nonetheless, for all practical purposes it can be accepted that attempting to form and change attitudes remains a worthwhile pursuit of those who wish to influence health-related behaviour.

Theories relevant to the formation of attitudes

Since persuasive communication still may be legitimately concerned with attitude change or attitude formation it is necessary to examine the contribution of some major theories to ideas about how attitudes are formed and changed.

1. Associative learning theories

Associative learning theories (which are described in Ch. 3) would suggest that attitudes are changed as individuals respond to rewards and punishments. Thus, the principles of classical and instrumental conditioning may be applied to attitude formation and change. Learning to associate positive and negative attitudes with a given health behaviour is assumed to be what motivates the individual to adopt or reject the behaviour. For instance, in dental health education it is common to concentrate upon the aesthetic aspects of good teeth, on the assumption that a person who believes good teeth are attractive will develop positive attitudes to teeth care.

2. Functional theories

Functional theories emphasise the relationship of persuasive communication to the person's underlying personality and motivational needs. Katz (1960) proposed that attitudes may serve four functions for the individual:

Instructional function : to satisfy needs, physical, social, emotional and intellectual;

Ego defence function : to protect the self-image, help the individual deal with conflicts;

Value expressive function : to give expression to self-concept and self-identity;

Knowledge function : to give meaning, by providing the individual with order and stability.

Other needs have been suggested, but all functionalists suggest that attitudes emerge to meet personal or social needs and that attitudes change when they are no longer functional. If this is applied, then it can be seen that according to functional theory a communication will persuade by addressing the issue of the function of the attitude to be changed. For instance, take the example of a man who needs to feel superior towards women and holds a belief that women are inferior drivers, based on that need. Factual information, even the best-researched evidence, will be unlikely to change his attitude to women drivers. In this case, persuasion will depend upon being able to help him identify and remove his need to feel superior.

3. Perceptual theories

Perceptual theories suggest that how the individual perceives a communication will affect whether or not he is persuaded by it. There are two main ways in which perception is said to exercise its effects (Sherif & Cantril, 1945, 1946). One is *selective perception* which implies that the individual selects the parts of the communication to which he will pay attention. The other is *frame of reference* which suggests that the context in which a message is received will influence how the individual reacts to it. In regard to attitude change, one perceptual theory of particular note is *Social Judgement Theory* (Sherif & Hovland, 1961). This suggests that the individual evaluates all incoming information and has a mechanism for acceptance or rejection based on existing personal latitudes of acceptance and rejection. If a message is judged to be within the *latitude of acceptance*, attitude change in response to communication will occur. If, however, the message is considered to fall within the *latitude of rejection*, either there is no attitude change or attitude change in the opposite direction to the position indicated in the message. Theories of perception explain the common finding of many persuasive communicators that people take what they want out of a message and that they listen best to things they want to hear. Hence the old saying that it is easier to preach to the converted.

4. Consistency theories

Consistency theories propose that the individual will strive to keep harmony within his internal belief system and that attitude change results from the need to make adjustments to restore or maintain harmony. That is, attitudes change when some fact, behaviour or event causes inconsistency or imbalance within the belief system. One theory which has applied the idea of balance to identifying what occurs in persuasion is *Congruity Theory* (Osgood & Tannenbaum, 1955). This suggests that if someone has a positive attitude towards a person and a negative attitude to a particular event or object he is likely to draw those two attitudes together if he finds out that the person he admires feels positively towards the event or idea he dislikes. He will either develop a less favourable attitude to the person or a more favourable attitude to the event or idea. In other words, he will shift his attitudes to make them more congruent. The theory predicts that if attitude change is necessary to restore congruity then both attitudes will change, the more extreme attitude changing least. Congruity theory, then, suggests that having a high regard for a message communicator may influence the person to change his attitudes, provided his positive attitude to the communicator is stronger than his negative attitudes to the position advocated. If someone feels strongly about a particular issue and his views clash with the advocate of that position, it is possible that he will review his opinion of the individual concerned, if that is the less strongly held attitude.

In general, consistency theories predict that the more a person likes the communicator the more likely he is to adopt attitudes held by the communicator. The exception to this is Festinger's (1957, 1964) *Cognitive Dissonance Theory.* This predicts that if individuals consider that they have voluntarily chosen to expose themselves to a persuasive communication, then they will change their attitudes when they dislike, rather than like, the source. This is a because the individual will tend to justify the decision to listen to someone he considers unworthy of his attention by believing that the message had intrinsic worth.

FACTORS AFFECTING COMMUNICATION AND PERSUASION

Communication in nursing care, whether or not it is intended to be persuasive, is influenced by a number of factors: the setting, the nurse, the patient or client and the message.

The setting

Picture a crowded, noisy room filled with people and smoke. How easy will it be to carry on a conversation in such a room? While the ideal situation would be the calm and quiet of a private room, the reality is that often nurses communicate with patients in their homes where children may be running about and playing, in hospital wards where the corner of the day room may be the only suitable venue, or in busy Accident and Emergency departments. However, some aspects of all environments can be considered for control:

1. *The noise level.* As far as possible the setting should be quiet so that the noise is not distracting the patient. Turn

down television sets, ask others in the vicinity to speak quietly, give children a quiet game or task such as reading or jigsaw puzzles.

   2. *The presence of others.* While a private room is desirable, when one is not available, keep the voice low and make it clear to the others in the room that, for a particular period, one patient only is to be the focus of attention. This will help to avoid interruption.

   3. *The arrangement of furniture.* Is the patient in bed? Does the placement of furniture allow for face-to-face positioning and eye-to-eye contact? Are there physical barriers between the participants? Are the participants comfortable?

   4. *Other environmental considerations.* Is there anything about the lighting which will detract from the communication process. For example, is the lighting adequate, allowing for assessment of nonverbal cues, or does it flicker and become an irritant? Are there other distractions such as lurid wall colours or too many posters and pictures?

The nurse

As a planned process, therapeutic and persuasive communication are controlled, to a large extent, by the nurse. Therefore, her skills and knowledge are crucial to the outcome. To develop competence it is necessary to check on personal skills and attitudes before and after each interaction. With experience this monitoring may be done throughout a communication session. Whilst acquiring communication skills, a simple self-check may be useful (see Table 4.2 for a version of a self-check).

Table 4.2 Self check on nursing communication skills

Was the language I used at the right level?
Did I meet the other person's needs or mine?
Did I adapt messages to verbal and non-verbal cues?
Did I provide useful written back-up material?
Did I listen?
Did I use questions well?
How did I deal with silences?
Did I accept or reject views opposing mine?

Empathy, respect for others and warmth have been noted as important characteristics of the successful therapeutic communicator (Gazda et al, 1975). An empathetic nurse is able to understand the feelings of the patient, to see things through his eyes. Sympathising, or actually having the same feelings, is a different characteristic which may prevent the patient from expressing himself fully and switch the focus to the nurse. Empathy is helpful and conducive to developing a therapeutic relationship. The following conversation excerpt illustrates degrees of empathy:

> *Patient* (a woman in hospital who is 4 days post-hysterectomy and is worrying about her 4 children at home): 'I do hope my husband is able to cope with them. They are such energetic children.'
>
> *Response 1*: *Nurse*: 'Four children can be a handful. I should know, I have 6!' (This response is not particularly helpful as the nurse did not acknowledge the worry factor and she turned the focus to herself).
>
> *Response 2*: *Nurse*: 'You sound a bit worried about your husband coping. Four children can be a handful. Has he spoken of how he's getting along at home?' (Here the nurse attends to the content: 4 children, husband having to cope; and the feeling: the worry).

Respecting others is synonymous with valuing and having confidence in others. As a health teacher the nurse must hold this position sincerely or the patient will not feel able to participate, to make decisions or to act on them. Being non-judgemental and accepting the person as he is allows the patient to be himself and to self-explore. A non-directive approach on the part of the nurse helps to convey this attitude of respect: 'I know you can do it, I'm here to help you find the best way possible for you.'

Besides having empathy and respect for the patient, the nurse also must develop a warmth which says to the patient that she is there to help, that she wants to help and that she cares about him and his situation. Nonverbal communication skills such as making eye contact, appearing relaxed and ready to listen indicate that the nurse has heard both the content and the feeling in what the patient says.

Table 4.3 summarises the points made about empathy, respect and warmth by listing some communication tips.

Credibility may sometimes be important, particularly if

Table 4.3 Some tips for therapeutic communication

Do	Don't
—establish a trust relationship	—be glib
—allow the patient the freedom to participate	—make premature judgements
—be helpful	—be opinionated
—set up a conducive atmosphere	—belittle
—regard the information as confidential	—change the subject

there is a need to persuade or give advice. Experiments have shown that people are more likely to be persuaded by a message if the source seems credible to them. To be accepted as credible, the communicator has to be acknowledged as having expertise and being trustworthy. In early explorations on the idea of credibility Hovland & Weiss (1951) demonstrated that the *New England Journal of Medicine* was more persuasive than a monthly picture magazine in discussing the advisability of selling antihistamine drugs without prescription. Presumably this is because doctors are regarded as having expert knowledge about drugs and a professional journal is therefore more persuasive than one generally intended for lay people. In some instances, credibility depends upon having relevant experience. Levine & Valle (1975) found that former alcoholics were more influential than others in changing students' attitudes about alcoholism, and McPeek & Edwards (1975) demonstrated that long-haired males were more persuasive in arguing against marijuana.

Credibility produces attitude change by a process Kelman (1961) labelled *internalisation*. This means that the new attitude becomes part of the individual's own value or belief system. Once new beliefs are internalised, they tend to be firmly held, even if the source changes stance on the issue.

Another aspect of source credibility which should be noted is the *sleeper effect*. This is so called because a number of studies have shown that low credibility sources appear to increase their impact after a time lapse. Why this should be so has not been established, but some researchers have suggested that because the source has low credibility the recipient is more likely to question the original message. Active involvement in producing counter-arguments causes the individual to examine his existing belief system, and convinces him of the validity of the position he eventually adopts.

Attractiveness of the source of a message also influences whether or not it will be well received. People are more likely to adopt attitudes of those they find likeable. Response to source attractiveness is said to happen in order to enhance self-concept. This process Kelman (1961) labelled *identification*. In this instance the individual will accept the attitude without internalising it. However, to maintain such an attitude the influence of the source must be continued. Once the source of influence is removed the attitude may be changed quite readily. Also, if the communicator's attitude changes, the recipient's will also be likely to change.

Whereas attitude change by internalisation usually depends upon verification of information being presented, change by identification is not dependent upon the validity of the position held nor upon the existence of evidence to support it. Norman (1976) demonstrated that a communicator was equally persuasive to groups whether or not he presented any reasons supporting the opinion that people sleep more than they need to.

Source attractiveness would appear to be a somewhat tenuous means of persuasion. Yet widespread use of communicator attractiveness is made in health education, as demonstrated by the use of sports and other media personalities in promoting positive health images. One reason for this is that it is often the case that attractive sources are characterised by skills and attributes which make them especially persuasive people. It is possible, therefore, that attractive sources change attitudes by internalisation as well as by identification, and this assumption underlies the widespread use of 'personalities' or image-sellers.

Power in the communicator brings about attitude change by a process Kelman (1961) termed *compliance*. He proposed that when a communicator has a powerful position in respect to the person receiving the message, there will be a tendency for the recipient to adopt the communicator's position publicly, but reject it privately. Power is exercised by the use of reward or punishment. In nursing settings it is not difficult to imagine that some clients or patients may feel vulnerable and respond to a powerful health care professional by wishing to please or to avoid incurring displeasure. Power exercised in this way can be very successful in achieving persuasion, but the results are likely to be shortlived once the powerful influence is removed. This may be one explanation of the repeated finding that patients fail to continue with a prescribed medical regimen once they leave hospital.

Psychologists studying persuasion use the word compliance in this quite specific sense. The term compliance is also used widely by nurses and doctors, but here the intended meaning is different. In medical and nursing terms the word compliance is used to indicate continued adherence to medical and nursing recommendations. Much traditional patient education has been based upon the idea of achieving such adherence, and the use of the word compliance for a successful outcome has not necessarily been an indication that the intention was to bring about change by the exercise of power. Nonetheless, it is interesting to note the dangers of the exercise of power, as well as the shortlived effects. Today, it is less acceptable than previously that nurses and doctors tell people what is good for them, and increasingly the emphasis is upon releasing patient power and reducing professional power.

Similarity between sender and receiver also increases the likelihood that the message will persuade. The explanation for this may be quite simple, in that a similar source appears either credible or attractive or both.

Credibility, attractiveness and power are all important characteristics to consider in choosing an effective communicator. Clearly these factors are not always separable in practice; a doctor, for instance, may be a powerful source of communication by virtue of the expertise and trustworthiness which give him credibility. Nurses, on the other hand, may be attractive sources of communication because they are perceived as less technically educated than doctors and therefore more similar to lay people. On the other hand, that very feature may in some instances increase credibility because 'the nurse understands, her experience of life is like mine', or decrease credibility because 'the nurse understands my position, but does she really know about the medical facts?' So the communicator role is complex and there are no hard and fast rules. The most satisfying and potentially useful approach to communication is for the nurse to examine what she has to bring to the situation, identifying factors which are likely to be strengths and weaknesses in regard to the particular person with whom she is communicating, the nature of the message, and the setting in which communication takes place.

The patient or client

There are many features of the person which may affect the communication process. First, his *psycho-physiological state* is important. Can he participate or has he some condition such as deafness, being in a comatose state, or being catatonic which will severely limit, if not block, attempts at communication? The nurse's initial assessment of the patient will determine his psycho-physiological state. Factors to note are educational level, age, developmental state, and emotions. Second, what is his *perception of the nurse*? Does he see her as a helper or as a nuisance? Has he had previous experience of health care personnel which now leads him to distrust them? Does she have credibility, attractiveness and power which he acknowledges? Third, are there *sociocultural factors* of which to be aware before helping the patient? For instance, are there religious dietary rules the patient follows which might affect maintaining strict adherence to a low calorie diet? Even more important, and sometimes difficult to ascertain, are there sociocultural influences which direct the patient's values and attitudes and, therefore, affect his motivation towards learning new health behaviours? Fourth, are there *personality characteristics* which might affect communication? A helpless, chronically anxious person may be unable to self-explore to a depth which would encourage resolution of a problem, whereas a confident person who is used to taking risks may be highly motivated to try new health behaviours. Two particular aspects of personality have generally been considered to have an effect upon how the individual will respond to persuasive health messages. These are internal–external control and self-esteem. Some people are more confident than others in their ability to control the environment in which they live. This aspect of personality has been labelled *internal-external* control, or locus of control. Rotter (1954, 1966) proposes that people who are at the internal end of the control continuum believe that events occur as a consequence of their own actions and under their control. Those at the external end, on the other hand, believe that events are not related to their personal behaviour and are therefore beyond their control. Since persuasive communication is usually directed at the individual from an external source, it seems likely that persons who see themselves as in control of the environment will be less likely to be influenced by external factors. 'Internal'persons will, therefore, resist persuasion rather well. There is some substance to this idea, but equally, it is possible that people who do not see themselves as being in control see no point in any health-related action, since, after all, most things are outside their personal control.

Everyone holds a concept of self. Some people see themselves favourable, others less so. This evaluative aspect of self-concept is called *self-esteem*. Carl Rogers (1951, 1959) claimed that a favourable self-concept is a necessary condition for mental health. Knowing that other people think well of them seems important to most people. Psychologists have proposed that the seeking of positive comments from others motivates and directs human behaviour. Health educators utilising an educational model have attempted to capitalise on this phenomenon, by designing educational programmes intended to promote self-esteem. A recent curriculum development project for schools, entitled 'All About Me' exemplifies this approach (Schools Council Project 5–13, 1977).

There is a clear case within nursing for promoting self-esteem in patients and in clients. It is less clear, however, what part self-esteem plays in governing responses to persuasion. Personality appears to be interlinked with social, psychological and cultural factors in determining health-related behaviour.

The message

While this aspect of communication may seem straightforward, researchers have discovered that messages may have complex repercussions.

Both the nature and content of the message, as well as the style of presentation, affect the way in which it is processed by the recipient and the extent to which it will persuade. Factors of note in persuasive messages are:

One-sided versus two-sided arguments

Some research has been done on whether people are more easily persuaded if the message presents one or two sides of an argument. Hovland et al (1949) demonstrated that two-sided messages were more effective with better educated audiences, whilst less well educated people were more easily persuaded by one-sided messages. In practice, of course, what happens in laboratory-type conditions is of little real interest to the health educator, since it is hardly likely that anyone will be able to be kept free of contamination by other views in today's world. Sooner or later the health educator who presents only one side of the case will be discredited. Despite this obvious truth, there is a tendency often for professionals to attempt to package a simplistic message containing only part of the truth when communicating with people whom they perceive to be uneducated.

Repetition

There is good evidence that repetition of a message is in itself persuasive. Greater exposure to a message increases recall and attitude formation (Solomon, 1972). Advertisers make great efforts to take message exposure to saturation level, and this is why so many compaigns are so very expensive. However, the exact mechanism by which repetition operates is not known and it is as well to remember that some repetition is tiresome, and can generate negative reactions. What evidence there is would suggest that the greatest benefits of repetition will accrue where the message is complex and that repetition of simple messages, with the risk of 'overkill', should be avoided.

Fear arousal

A number of researchers have looked at whether fear will motivate people to take preventive action in relation to their health. Use of fear arousal as a health education technique is suggested on the grounds that people will be motivated to reduce the risk of developing a particular disease if they are presented with fear-producing information about the condition while at the same time being given reassuring advice about how to avoid it. For instance, the health educator might show pictures of gum disease and in the same lesson talk about the benefits and techniques of tooth-brushing.

Janis & Fesbach (1953) demonstrated that high fear appeals worked less well than low fear appeals in motivating people to adopt good dental hygiene practices. That finding cast doubt upon the use of fear arousal as a health education technique. Later studies, however, have shown that fear arousal may be effective in some circumstances. Leventhal (1970) provided a possible explanation of why the response to fear appeals varies. He proposed that fear arousal was likely to provoke two parallel responses in the individual: fear control and danger control. Individuals receiving fear arousing messages will be motivated to control fear as well as danger. In some circumstances, particularly in high threat, the need to control fear would outweigh the need to control danger and emotional response might just prevent the person from taking any action against the disease. It is possible, for instance, that fear arousal in breast cancer education might result in someone being afraid to find out she had the disease, and thus too afraid to present herself for mammography. Two studies have supported this proposition, by demonstrating that those who perceive themselves as at risk are less likely to be influenced to action by high fear appeals. Leventhal & Watts (1966) demonstrated this in regard to smokers' response to communication about lung cancer, and Berkowitz & Cottingham (1966) showed that fear appeals in relation to seat belt use were less effective with regular than occasional drivers. It seems that people who see themselves as vulnerable respond by controlling fear and the fear control response inhibits action to control the danger.

It is also possible that people with high self-esteem respond to fear appeals while people with low self-esteem do not. A study by Goldstein (1959) showed that people labelled as 'copers', confronted with a high fear arousal message and a specific plan of avoiding action, adopted the recommended action whilst those identified as 'avoiders' did not.

In general, it can be said that fear appeals work with some people and in some circumstances, but that it is difficult to predict the effects of arousing fear.

Message content

There has been less research in the area of message content than in other aspects of message effects such as fear appeal and one and two-sided messages. Fishbein & Ajzen (1981) have identified this as a serious omission, asserting that message content interacts with other effects in accomplishing persuasion. They argue that indirect effects of the message, in other words, the impact upon beliefs other than the ones to which the message is addressed, should be given special consideration when messages are designed. For instance, the claim that a detergent is powerful may cause housewives to react favourably to it because a powerful detergent may be expected to get the wash clean. However, some housewives may believe that powerful detergents harm clothes and this may generate a negative reaction to the message. Impact effects are clearly of importance in health teaching. Consider the impact on pregnant females who are smokers of the fact that smoking during pregnancy reduces birth weight: if they believe that low birth weight will be an advantage in labour or small babies are more attractive than heavy ones, then they are not likely to be discouraged from smoking. Fishbein & Ajzen also argue that there is little to gain from manipulating the factors which will increase attention to or understanding of the message, since some messages seem to be accepted without any supporting evidence: people do adopt new ideas without any detailed understanding of why they matter. This, however, seems more likely to be a consideration for the pure researcher or the propagandist than for the nurse as health teacher.

The interrelationship of sender–receiver message factors

Clearly, there are as many questions as answers arising from research in the field of persuasive communication. However, review of theories and experimental studies would suggest that the message is more likely to persuade if:

The source is   — credible
                   — attractive
                   — powerful
                   — similar to the recipient

The message is
— repeated
— promotes functional fear arousal
— is perceived as relevant
— is designed with consideration of the impact on a set of beliefs

The recipient
— has the 'right' personality *or*
— is helped to feel some self-esteem
— gains a sense of control over what is happening
— is challenged and supported as he processes new information

What individual studies fail to illuminate is whether or how such factors are interrelated.

In persuasive communication the central question of what motivates the health-related actions of an individual remains. Rosenstock (1974) records that early research attempts to explain why individuals take or avoid preventive health action evolved the *Health Belief Model*. The original model proposed that the combined effect of an individual's perception of the severity of a disease and his own susceptibility to it would provide the energy or force to act to prevent the disease, provided he was sufficiently convinced that the prescribed course of action would be beneficial and worth his personal trouble and costs. Becker (1974) has provided a collection of papers which record how the model was tested and evolved. The model posed questions about the role of beliefs about susceptibility, seriousness and perceived benefits in motivating preventive health actions, and provided for examination of ways in which factors such as age, sex, race, ethnicity, personality, social class, peer pressure and knowledge from various sources would interrelate to increase or decrease the likelihood of the individual taking preventive health action. In commenting upon the state of research related to the role of beliefs in motivating health actions, Kirscht (1974) has suggested that the various testings of the Health Belief Model do substantiate the idea that beliefs energise and direct behaviour. What is not as yet known, however, is which set of beliefs is sufficient to predict or direct any given behaviour, and what processes enter into belief change in relation to behaviour. Despite all the work that has been done, research on modifying beliefs and behaviour has hardly scratched the surface.

In the circumstances, the best the practising health educator can do is provide a check list of possible beliefs and the psychosocial and cultural factors which seem likely to militate for or against the proposed action by the person, and keep these in mind when assessing teaching needs. The application of this approach is demonstrated in Chapter 6.

REFERENCES

Ajzen I, Fishbein M 1977 Attitude—behaviour relations: a theoretical analysis and review of empirical research, Psychological Bulletin 84: 888–918
Argyle M 1975 Bodily communication. Methuen, London
Becker M H (ed) 1974 The health belief model and personal health behaviour. Charles B Slack Inc, Thorofare, New Jersey
Berkowitz L, Cottingham D R 1960 The interest value and relevance of fear arousing communications. Journal of Abnormal and Social Psychology 60: 37–43
Festinger L 1957 A theory of cognitive dissonance. Stanford University Press, Stanford, California
Festinger L 1964 Conflict decision and dissonance. Stanford University Press, Stanford, California
Fishbein M, Ajzen I 1981 Acceptance yielding and impact: cognitive processes in persuasion. In: Petty R E, Ostram T M, Brock T C (eds) Cognitive responses in persuasion. Lawrence Erlbaum Associates, Hillsdale, New Jersey
Garrett A 1972 Interviewing, its principles and methods, 2nd edn. Family Service Association of America, New York
Gazda G M, Walters R P, Childers W C 1975 Human relations development: a manual for health sciences. Allyn & Bacon, London
Goldstein M J 1959 The relationship between coping and avoiding behaviour and response to fear arousing propaganda. Journal of Abnormal and Social Psychology 58: 247–252
Hargie O, Saunders C, Dickson D 1981 Social skills in interpersonal communication, Croom Helm, London
Hein E C 1980 Communication in nursing practice, 2nd edn. Little, Brown & Co, Boston
Hovland C I, Lumsdaine A A, Sheffield F D 1949 Experiments on mass communication. Princeton University Press, Princeton, New Jersey
Hovland C I, Weiss W 1951 The influence of source credibility on communication effectiveness. Public Opinion Quarterly 15: 635–650
Janis I L, Fesbach S 1953 Effects of fear arousing communications. Journal of Abnormal and Social Psychology 48: 78–92
Katz D 1960 The functional approach to the study of attitudes. Public Opinion Quarterly 24 (Summer):163–204
Kelman H 1961 Processes of opinion change. Public Opinion Quarterly 25: 57–58
Kreiger D, Peper E, Ancoli S 1979 Therapeutic touch, searching for evidence of physiological change. American Journal of Nursing 79 (April): 660–662

Kirsht J P 1974 Research related to the modification of health beliefs. In: Becker M H (ed) The health belief model and personal health behaviour. Charles B Slack Inc, Thorofare, New Jersey

La Piere R T 1934 Attitudes versus actions. Social Forces 13: 230–237

Leventhal H 1970 Findings and theory in the study of fear communications. In: Berkowitz L (ed) Advances in experimental social psychology 5. Academic Press, New York

Leventhal H, Watts J C 1966 Sources of resistance to fear arousing communications on smoking and lung cancer. Journal of Personality 34: 155–175

Levine J M, Valle R S 1975 The convert as a credible source. Social behaviour and personality 3(1): 81

McPeek R W, Edwards J D 1975 Expectancy, disconfirmation and attitude change. Journal of Social Psychology 96(2): 193–207

Mason A, Pratt J 1980 Touch. Nursing Times 76(3): 999–1001

Norman R 1976 When what is said is important: a comparison of expert and attractive sources. Journal of Experimental Psychology 12: 294–300

Osgood C E, Tannenbaum P H 1955 The principle of congruity in the prediction of attitude change. Psychological Review 62: 42–55

Petty R E, Ostram T M, Brock T C (eds) 1981 Cognitive responses in persuasion. Lawrence Erlbaum Associates, Hillsdale, New Jersey

Rogers C R 1951 Client centred therapy: its current practice implications and theory. Houghton Mifflin, Boston

Rogers C R 1959 A theory of therapy personality and interpersonal relationships as developed in a client centred framework. In: Koch S (ed) Psychology: a study of science, vol 3. McGraw Hill, New York

Rosenstock I M 1974 Historical origins of the health belief model. In: Becker M H (ed) The health belief model and personal health behaviour. Charles B Slack Inc, Thorofare, New Jersey

Rotter J B 1954 Social learning and clinical psychology. Prentice Hall, Englewood Cliffs, New Jersey

Rotter J B 1966 Generalised expectations for internal versus external control of reinforcement. Psychological Monographs 80(1): 1–28

Sherif M, Cantril H 1945 The psychology of attitudes 1. Psychological Review 52: 295–319

Sherif M, Cantril H 1946 The psychology of attitudes 11. Psychological Review 53: 1–24

Sherif M, Hovland C 1961 Social judgement: assimilation and contrast effects in communication and attitude change. Yale University Press, New Haven, Conn.

Solomon H 1972 The effects of multiple exposure source credibility and initial option on communication effectiveness. Dissertation Abstracts International 33(3-A):1227

FURTHER READING

Argyle M 1981 Social skills and health. Methuen, London

Hein E C 1980 Communication in nursing practice, 2nd ed. Little, Brown & Co, Boston

Morris D 1977 Manwatching: a field guide to human behaviour. Jonathan Cape, London

Mostyn B 1978 The attitude behaviour relationship. MCB Publications. Yorkshire

Teaching techniques for
   cognitive learning
Teaching techniques for
   affective learning

Teaching techniques for
   skills learning
Choosing teaching
   techniques and aids

5

Teaching techniques and aids

OBJECTIVES

Study of this chapter will enable you to:

1. Discuss factors involved in increasing recall and understanding.
2. Identify a range of teaching techniques and aids suitable for health teaching.
3. Discuss the advantages and limitations of each of the techniques and aids.
4. Identify teaching strategies which enhance different kinds of learning.
5. Select appropriate teaching methods and materials for a range of situations in which nurses teach about health.

TEACHING TECHNIQUES FOR COGNITIVE LEARNING

One of the tasks of the health teacher is to present information effectively. Being able to do this depends upon selecting those teaching strategies and aids which will encourage and stimulate recall and understanding.

Factors which influence recall and understanding

One of the main barriers to communication between professionals and lay people is that many people are unfamiliar
with the *technical language* which nurses and doctors use
everyday. There are two ways to tackle the problem. Sometimes lay terms can be substituted for technical ones, thus
setting the person at ease. Having a familiar starting point facilitates the absorption of new material. The other approach
is to use the technical term and to explain its meaning. Generally this is more useful because it may help the person in
future communications with other health care professionals.
Access to technical language can be a decided asset to patients, helping them to achieve partnership in communication.

That people without a facility for technical language can be
at a disadvantage was demonstrated some time ago in a study
of communication between general practitioners and patients
(Pratt et al, 1957). 89 general practitioners were observed communicating with 214 patients. All of the doctors tended to un-
derestimate the patients' knowledge. Those they perceived as
particularly poorly informed received less information than
those they thought were quite well informed. A curious
vicious circle was observed. The doctor arbitrarily assessed a
given patient and assumed he would have little or no technical
language. He then avoided using such language during the
consultation and made no attempt at dealing with any complex issues because of his conviction that the patient would
not understand in any case. In turn the patient, sensitive to
a lack of information being offered by the doctor, responded
by not asking any questions.

In talking with people about health it is important to avoid
using jargon which may alienate. Nonetheless, using and explaining technical terms may be a great help in reducing people's dependency upon health care professionals. In general,
younger and more educated people will understand more
technical language, but even here assumptions should be
avoided. It is always best to ask the person what things mean
to him, since sometimes lay and professional people use the
same terms but with different meanings.

It is also worthwhile to remember that there is a limit to
everyone's memory, thus the *amount of information* to be

given must be considered carefully. On average people will remember two out of six statements given at any one time and the more information that is given the greater the proportion of it which will be forgotten. Ley & Spelman (1967) have described a series of experiments which would suggest that the only way to be reasonably sure people will remember all that they are told is to give only two items of information at a time. This has obvious implications for health teaching in hospital, where it has been common practice to produce a diet of facts on admission and just prior to discharge. This almost guarantees that the person will forget most of what he has been told because it is humanly impossible to absorb the amount of material presented in the time allowed. It is very important, in any health teaching setting, to make arrangements to present information in small amounts at appropriate intervals.

The *sequencing of information items* also has an impact upon recall and understanding. Experimental studies (Ley & Spelman, 1967) have shown that two main features influence which information items are remembered best: the position of the item in the sequence and how important it is perceived to be. In general, it can be assumed that people will remember, most consistently, the first item in any series of items presented. They are also more likely to be able to recall items they consider to be important. Ley & Spelman (1965) demonstrated that hospital outpatients remembered diagnostic statements and those giving information about their illness better than statements about investigation or instructions for care. It is reasonably certain, therefore, that if diagnosis is the first item of information given it will be remembered. Clearly, it is important for the person to know his diagnosis. Often, however, there is equal concern to have him remember details of treatment and self-care. Indeed, knowledge of diagnosis may be of little value if he has not grasped how his condition may be managed and the part he must play in management. In theory, the way round this situation might be to give instructions first and diagnosis last, thus enhancing the chance of instructions being remembered. In practice this option makes little sense. People expect to know what is wrong with them. They are likely to feel anxious and entitled to be aggrieved if they think that information is being withheld. When instructions are important, information-giving sessions should be structured so that details of diagnosis and instructions are separated. There is great advantage in giving the person time to come to terms with his diagnosis before presenting him with details of his self-care.

One way of getting around the problem of too many items, perhaps of equal importance, is to *structure the information* in some way. Most people remember best, information they are able to categorise or organise for themselves. Hence the general popularity of mnemonics and other aids to memory. It may help therefore to categorise the information for people and to indicate the number of items to be remembered in each category. For instance, a message to a hospital inpatient might be structured: 'I am going to tell you about your diagnosis, the results of the investigations done while you have been in hospital, and about your treatment. Firstly, about your diagnosis there are two things to say . . .', and so on. Ley (1973) considerably increased the ability of both student volunteers and general practice patients to recall 15 statements presented to them by letting them know in advance what categories of information would be presented and by careful choice of the sequence of items.

By far the most common reason for advice to be forgotten is that it is *insufficiently specific*. A general exhortation to 'take it easy' means something different to almost everyone who hears it. What would be slowing down for some people represents increased activity for others. General statements are neither convincing nor helpful, and people promptly forget what they find difficult to interpret. Bradshaw et al (1975) have demonstrated experimentally that advice is more likely to be recalled if it is specific, while a series of experiments described by Ley (1976) showed that improved readability together with categorisation of information items and specificity can increase the effectiveness of a patient education leaflet. In one of these experiments, leaflets were used to assist people to lose weight. It was found that an experimental group exposed to a specifically designed leaflet lost considerably more weight than a control group exposed to a standard leaflet.

In some situations, for instance in relation to exercise or drug therapy, it is necessary to be very specific indeed, quite simply because the person may not have enough background information to be able to interpret instructions. Riley (1966) constructed a list of instructions he thought patients might find difficult to follow. It contained statements such as: avoid foods containing starch and sugar, avoid substances containing aspirin, decrease salt as much as possible, avoid fatty foods, and so on. He then devised a multiple choice questionnaire designed to test whether patients would have enough information to interpret such general instructions and demonstrated that a large proportion of general practice patients did not. Thus, following a prescribed regime in these cases probably met with a low success rate.

It can be very difficult to find sufficient opportunities to allow each person to learn at his own pace. One solution to this is to provide *written reminders* of factual material. A list of instructions helps the person remember what he has been asked to do. It also helps relatives who may be involved in assisting with self-care in a period of recovery. If the instructions are complex, illustrations may be needed.

It is important that any written instructions are presented in language which is understood easily. Educational psychologists have evolved a number of tests of readability. These usually consist of applying a simple formula to sample passages from the written material concerned. In general, they examine sentence length and numbers of syllables, since these have been identified as factors influencing readability. Short sentences and few syllables is a good general rule.

One simple but effective way of ensuring that the patient understands written instructions is to involve him in writing them. It can be very helpful to encourage patients to take notes while instructions are given and to discuss them afterwards. In addition to leaving the patient with a reminder he will understand, this method ensures his involvement, assisting both memory and motivation.

The *immediate personal experience* of the patient, factors such as anxiety or pain, may impair his usual ability to understand or recall information. Important instructions should therefore be timed carefully, and repeated as necessary. Though it may be helpful to outline post-operative care preoperatively, it is unrealistic to expect anyone to remember details at a time of high anxiety. Clearly, it will be necessary to repeat some information. It may even be helpful to withhold unnecessary detail of post-operative progress until after surgery has taken place. Similarly, someone in acute pain immediately after admission with myocardial infarction should not be subjected to any more detail than is necessary. It is not always easy to judge how much information patients want, and when is the best time to give it. Some people, even in considerable pain or distress will indicate verbally or otherwise that they want to know what is likely to happen to them, and what treatments will be undertaken. Information should never be withheld, though many people may be satisfied with quite brief answers in the first instance if they are assured that an opportunity to discuss detail will be forthcoming. That assurance will not be supplied by evasiveness and a promise to tell later, but rather by an obvious willingness to listen and to supply information as and when the person indicates a desire for it.

All of these factors—the use of technical language; the amount of information and its sequence, organisation and specificity; the use of written reminders; and consideration of the immediate personal experience of the learner—are important considerations when trying to increase recall and understanding.

The lecture method

Cognitive aspects of learning are concerned with the way the individual processes information in order to understand and remember it. Nurses often present information to patients or clients on an individual basis, but sometimes a number of people have to be taught the same things. In such cases nurses give *lectures* or talks to groups. The lecture is a traditional teaching technique which offers a useful way of presenting learners with a framework of what is to be learned.

Format and use of the lecture

In health teaching a lecture should be no longer than 15 or 20 minutes and it should be tightly organised with a clear cut beginning and end. The normal format is to introduce oneself, if necessary, and the object of the lecture; give a brief outline of the content and describe the format of the session; give the lecture; summarize the session; and, thank the learners for their attention. In some situations it may be helpful to give a written reminder of what has been said. The lecture can be used with other methods. For example, it could introduce a series of sessions on preparation for childbirth. A short talk is often a very welcome beginning to a new course as not everyone will want to plunge into discussion straight away. An introductory outline of material will often alert listeners to items they may raise in discussion later. Despite changes in teaching methods in schools, there is still widespread acceptance of the idea that in a teaching session the teacher will do the talking. While it will be useful to establish later that all group members have a role to play in exploring health issues, having the teacher speak first is often a reassuring beginning.

Delivery of the lecture is very much a matter of personal style; some mannerisms add to the speaker's attractiveness, others detract. There are a number of 'dos and don'ts': do move while lecturing but don't pace; do scan all the faces in the audience; don't use 'um' or 'er' frequently; do be well prepared so as to avoid embarrassing pauses, and do not use the blackboard frequently, otherwise the learners will view mostly the lecturer's back. Blackboard material should be meticulous and easy to read. Use of notes is a good idea because they help maintain a cogent argument and prevent too many irrelevant anecdotes. On the other hand, it is important to maintain a reasonably lively delivery and so reading verbatim should be avoided. It may be best to speak to annotated headings rather than to have the talk written out in full. The lecture should be given within the allotted time which means keeping an eye on a watch or clock. Beyond the scheduled time the attention span of the listeners will begin to waver. Once started, the lecturer should check that her voice can be heard.

Limitations. It is wise to remember that a lecture presents the information in the same manner to all those who are listening, whatever their needs, and since people process information differently and absorb new details at varying paces, some people may learn very little. The lecture method, therefore, has limitations in health teaching and should not be the only method of choice if the intention is to help people explore thinking and examine attitudes. Keeping the initial talk to 20 minutes or less and following with an opportunity for questions, helps to overcome some of the shortcomings of the lecture method. Alternatively, when a teaching session is to last an hour or so, it may be possible to arrange for material to be presented in three 10-minute sessions interspaced with opportunities for the group to ask questions and discuss. Again, this is a good way to begin a series of lessons because the initial questions and discussion help the teacher to appraise the level of knowledge and type of teaching required and thus to make immediate adjustments to the learners' needs.

Generating questions. It will be necessary to have a strategy for coping with the silence which almost inevitably falls when the first opportunity to ask questions is given. There are two main reasons for silence. The first is that people need time to formulate questions. It is important to relax and wait and so make time available; there is always a temptation to dash in with something to fill the void. In health teaching this is particularly counterproductive because nurses are often asked to teach people with whom they have relatively limited contact and questions may be the best clue available to the real learning needs. The second reason for the initial silence may be that the majority of people in the group find it difficult to ask questions: they may be afraid to expose ignorance; have little experience of speaking up in a group of people; or, they may consider that questioning may be interpreted as challenging the teacher's authority. Again, this can be overcome by waiting in a relaxed manner and by reducing any threat in the way the question is asked. The bold 'Are there any questions?' may be substituted by, 'I'll stop now and give you a chance to say something . . .' or such prompts as, 'Have any of you had the experience of . .?', 'What do you think of this (picture, idea, etc.)?' and so on. The first question or comment from the group will usually open up a floodgate of others. Questions should be responded to positively as this invites further risk-taking on the part of the listeners. Starting a reply by saying something like 'I'm glad you asked that . . .' acknowledges and appreciates the participation.

TEACHING TECHNIQUES FOR AFFECTIVE LEARNING

Since attitudes and beliefs are formed in a social context, they are best examined in relation to other people. Sometimes feelings also need to be shared and explored with others and so group work is an important method in relation to affective learning.

Group work

Grouping people to listen to a lecture, even when they have maximum opportunity to ask questions, is not what is meant by group teaching. Nor is a group automatically formed because the number of people present is small or because seating has been arranged in a circle or semi-circle instead of in rows facing front.

Effective group work requires several persons to work and learn together. The presence of other group members and their contributions helps one to consider and respond to their feelings, ideas and opinions. Group work promotes recognition of similarities and differences. One can learn how to participate in the group, thereby increasing interaction skills.

Group work in health teaching depends upon the assumption that a group has certain basic characteristics which will facilitate expression of feelings, sharing of ideas and exploration of attitudes and beliefs. In some professional settings, for instance social work and psychiatry, group work is used as a therapeutic tool. In health teaching, group work is used as an educational tool and the health educator will normally neither have nor exercise the skills of a therapist in respect of the exploration of values and feelings. There is an obvious exception to this in the case of psychiatric nursing, but that is beyond the scope of this text.

Group characteristics

Any group has a number of common characteristics:

1. Definable membership. A group will have at least two members and they will be distinguished by name or type. For instance, a set of student nurses, a class of prenatal mothers, and a self-help organisation such as Alcoholics Anonymous are all groups.

2. *Common identity*. Members of a group have a sense of belonging to the group; they consciously identify with one another.

3. *Interdependence and common goals*. A gathering of people arrives at group feeling when they have the same goals or ideals and when they know thay have to depend upon each other to achieve those goals or meet needs. For example, people in pressure groups need each other because collective action will achieve their ends. They associate willingly because they share the same aspirations for change. Likewise, in self-help groups people are conscious that the help of others is necessary to meet their needs, for example for support while stopping smoking.

4. *Interaction*. When a group has formed, the members communicate with one another; they will respond to the views of others and be influenced by others in the group.

5. *Working as one*. In some indefinable way a group, once formed, takes on its own life and energy. Individuals in the group learn to make their contribution in a way that enables the group to work together, so that the group somehow behaves as a single organism.

Obviously there are many different kinds of groups, more than ever in today's society, but all of them will display, to greater or lesser extent, these basic characteristics.

Use of groups in health teaching

Nurses will operate as health teachers with two types of group: those whose primary purpose is other than health learning, for instance, a Women's Guild, or Parent Teachers' Association; and those specially convened for the purpose of learning about health, such as patients having pre-operative teaching, groups learning about child rearing, members of the public who have responded to an advertisement offering help to stop smoking or teaching about alcohol and alcoholism. In either case, group work is used because the process of working in a group has something to offer those who need to learn about their health.

The origins of group use in health education lie in experimental work done in the 1940s by Lewin (1947) who used group process to assist in such activities as motivating women to introduce offal to the family diet or giving babies orange juice. Lewin demonstrated that the group provided a persuasive force. Housewives in his studies were more persuaded to change by group sessions than by lectures because there was discussion of the problems involved in the change. Having to make and announce a decision and being able to see what other people had decided were also persuasive factors. Generally speaking, individuals are motivated to conform to a group decision to the extent that they need the approval and acceptance of the group.

Use of groups within health teaching has grown as ideas about health education options have developed. Nowadays, health teachers still use groups to persuade people to change attitudes. Equally, group work is used to reduce the authority dependence generated by traditional health education approaches, and groups may be set up on an entirely self-directed model on the assumption that the health educator's role is to enable rather than to persuade.

Preparing for group work

In planning to use a group for teaching purposes there are a number of things to consider which may influence the dynamics of group work:

1. Background. If the group is a new one people will have to get to know each other or find ways of working together. If members are similar to one another in respect of abilities, attitudes and aptitudes as well as social status, group work will usually be enhanced.

The established existence of a group means that the members may have no need to clarify the task before them. They will already have ways of working together. Some established groups have ways of working together which will assist the health teaching process. Others may have developed habits which hinder; for instance, some groups get used to having only a few people speak up or they may argue a lot.

2. Expectations. Groups who invite outside experts such as nurses to teach them have a variety of expectations. Some will want to participate in group work, others may anticipate receiving a lecture. Sometimes the group has existing behavioural constraints which make establishing group work very difficult. People who are used to having the teacher do all the leading and talking and be the person with ideas may find it very threatening to be expected to participate.

3. Size. A small group may increase participation and consensus but more members means more resources, more ideas and the task may be accomplished in a shorter period of time. An intermediate size of around 10 members should draw on the positive aspects of both small and large groups and encourage discussion without threat.

4. Cohesiveness. While it is important that the group members feel close, if they are too closely knit, this aspect becomes dysfunctional. The group needs to be open to new information and ideas. Co-operation and open communication promote a healthy level of cohesiveness.

5. Environment. Groups generally benefit from feeling that they have a place of their own in which to meet. If all goes well in a group than the members will arrange the environment to suit themselves. For the first meeting, however, it may help to arrange chairs so that people can see and hear each other and to minimise distractions (such as noise) from outside. Physical arrangements need to be reasonably good, but the most important environmental factor is the creation of a relaxed and friendly atmosphere in which people will learn to trust and respect each other.

6. Formation. As a group forms it may be observed going through a number of stages (see Fig. 5.1).

Group roles

In any group the roles assumed by both the leaders and the members are of paramount importance for they may influence the achievement of goals and objectives for each individual within the group.

Leadership roles in groups vary with the nature and purpose of the group. There is no set of functions which would be universally acknowledged to be the leader's role. However, the group usually does have expectations of the leader and

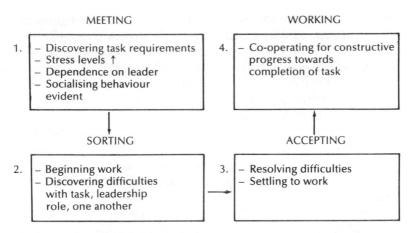

Figure 5.1 Four stages of group work

the style associated with that role. The style of leadership affects group process. There are teachers who want to control and to do things their way. Others allow members to decide how to proceed and thus their involvement equals that of other members. Still others allow students to 'do their own thing'. Whichever style is used or deliberately developed, the effects of it on group work should be evaluated.

Some now classic experiments on the effects of leadership style (White & Lippett, 1968) attempted to measure the effects of 3 different types of leadership behaviour: authoritarian, democratic and laissez-faire. Results showed that *authoritarian leadership*, where the leader took complete control of the group, increased the quantity and quality of work that the group could produce in the short term. However, group members demonstrated hostility to each other and to the leader, and there was aggression and competition. Also, groups led by authoritarian leaders were more discontented, developed dependence upon the leader and showed less originality. Groups working under *democratic leadership*, where the leader kept some control of the group, but encouraged involvement of members in deciding about group tests and methods, were much slower in producing work. They, however, appeared to be more motivated and their productivity increased as time went on. The atmosphere in these groups was friendly; members praised each other's efforts, worked as a team and were satisfied with the arrangements for the group. Under *laissez-faire leadership*, where the leader remained in the background and allowed group members to take all the initiative, less work was done and it was of poorer quality. Members were aggressive and fooled around more than in the other groups.

Clearly, for some groups, authoritarian leadership may be best, especially if there is a specific task to be completed in a short time. Generally speaking, however, the democratic style of leadership is more likely to be useful in health teaching since the aim is to increase independence in those being taught.

Member roles. Early work on group roles (Benne & Sheats, 1948) distinguished functions in relation, first, to group building and maintenance and, second, to group tasks.

Building and maintenance functions in groups were identified as the following:

Encouraging	: being friendly, responsive, praising, accepting contributions
Mediating	: conciliating, compromising
Gate-keeping	: facilitating contributions by others
Following	: being an audience, a good listener
Relieving tension	: draining off negative feelings by joking or clarifying the subject.

Group task functions included introducing new ways of looking at things, information-seeking and giving, opinion-giving, clarifying, elaborating and summarising. On that breakdown it is obvious that leadership and membership roles may be interchangeable.

Potential problems

In any group problems may arise. Usually these are related to self-centred behaviour of members. The following may need to be dealt with from time to time, either by the leader or by the group:

1. Obstructive moves to block progress. These may include going off at a tangent, rejecting ideas without consideration, arguing on a point everyone else has accepted. Obstructive members may withdraw from the activity by using deliberate silence or behaviour which indicates disinterest (yawning, talking to neighbours, doodling or resorting to excessive formality).

2. *Demands to meet personal needs.* These may include insisting on sharing personal experiences to the reduced participation of others; asking for help to draw attention to self or special pleading in the form of introduction of pet themes or claims to be speaking for the 'grass roots'.

3. *Excessive aggression and competition.* These may include criticising or blaming others, interrupting, taking over the discussion, referring only to the group leader, denigrating the contributions of others or asserting authority.

Every group member has a part to play in reducing potential problems, but clearly the leader has a special role to play in minimising self-centred behaviour in the group.

Monitoring group process

Groups form best and learn or work most when they are encouraged to monitor *process*, or what is going on in the group. In situations where there is clear intention to minimise the likelihood of dependency upon a professional health teacher, monitoring of group process will be particularly important and teaching group members to observe and record group process will be an essential part of the nurse's role.

The role of the observer in a group is to monitor and record what is going on, to interpret what is seen and heard and to report it to the group. The observer has to be able to give an honest account, including pointing out any problems which may be developing. The observer role is not as straightforward as it may seem, observers have to consider tone of voice as well as what is said and nonverbal, as well as verbal, behaviour. It requires skill to interpret behaviour without judging the person. A group needs feedback on group-building and maintenance, group progress towards accomplishing tasks, group style, and group interaction including self-orientated behaviour.

Process recording techniques. A technique useful for inexperienced observers is the sociogram. It requires mapping out the positions of group members and then drawing arrows to indicate the direction of any verbal interaction. Figure 5.2

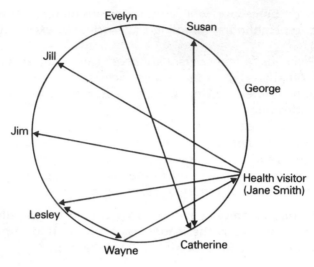

Figure 5.2 A sociogram representing a class of eight High School students who were discussing drug dependency in their city. The health visitor is acting as a facilitator to group discussion. The lines indicate the number of comments made in the 15 minutes the observer recorded. The arrows indicate the direction of the comments. For example, Jane Smith directed comments to Jill, Jim and Lesley. George was not involved at all. This analysis illustrates who spoke and to whom.

shows a sociogram drawn during the first few minutes of a discussion group looking at a drug problem. The person who records the sociogram should be asked to interpret it for the rest of the class and lead discussion on its interpretation. Another technique is to ask one or two members to note evidence of group building and maintenance of group task functions being undertaken, or self-centred behaviour displayed. People learning to observe should be briefed about their role (see Fig. 5.3 for a sample brief) and given a simple recording sheet to help them in their task (see Fig. 5.4 for example). It may be possible to arrange for the group to observe themselves, using video recording facilities.

TEACHING TECHNIQUES FOR SKILLS LEARNING

The theoretical framework for teaching skills comes from the two major areas of learning theory: association theories and

Observer's brief

Your role as observer is to give feedback to the group about how they are tackling their health learning or health-related problem.
Concentrate on what you see and hear people doing rather than what you *think* they may be feeling.
You are to note the *behaviour* of group members, and comment on individual contributions to group maintenance or group task functions. You should also record examples of self-centred behaviour.

Figure 5.3   Example of an observer's brief

Here is a list of behaviour observable in most groups:

Task functions	Group building	Self-centred behaviour
Initiating	Encouraging	Diverting the group
Information seeking	Compromising	Withdrawing
Information giving	Bringing others in	Interruption
Opinion giving	Setting standards	Denigrating others
Elaborating	Relieving tension	Rejecting ideas
Summarising	Listening	Dominating discussion

Note below examples of any of the above which you see during the group's work

Behaviour	By (Name)	To (Name)	Reminder notes

Figure 5.4   Example of a recording sheet used to analyse group member participation

cognitive theories. Association theories propose that learning occurs when a stimulus and a response become associated, usually by the application of reward or punishment. In health teaching, rewards are more usually applied than punishments. Rewards are provided by helping the individual to achieve

success; people are motivated by goals which make some demands but are not too daunting. One answer to the challenge
of teaching skills, therefore, would be to identify separate
manageable parts for the learner, and teach a little at a time.
Cognitive theories, on the other hand, suggest that learning
occurs when the individual sees the whole and grasps the relationship of parts, so that another possible approach to
teaching skills is to demonstrate the skilled performance and
thus allow the learner to see what he is aiming at. In practice,
most teachers combine these approaches, first demonstrating
the skill and its importance, and then assisting the learner to
identify and achieve the component parts.

[handwritten margin note: break it into stages]

Demonstration

Teaching new mothers how to bath baby is an example of a
demonstration commonly given by nurses. First the organisation of materials is shown, then the undressing of the baby
with discussion of the safety precautions such as the nappy
pins, keeping a steadying hand on the baby to prevent falling.
Later the bathing of the baby is done, demonstrating the 'top
to bottom', 'clean to unclean' principles. Finally, the end of
the demonstration includes drying and clothing the baby and
also care of the umbilical cord area. Frequently, this kind of
demonstration includes advice on nappy rash, checking the
fontanelle, and dry skin care. There is a great deal of useful
information which can be given, and mothers may feel over-
whelmed. A repeat demonstration in parts may be helpful:
(1) organisation of bath materials (2) handling and undressing
baby (3) bathing (4) after care. Time for discussion and feedback is essential. The need for repetition of the demonstration
followed by practice with supervision should be decided by
both mother and nurse. The extent of learning may be assessed through the repeated practice sessions.

Preparing a demonstration requires as much thought and
prior preparation as any other form of teaching. It should not
be assumed that the skilled performer will automatically demonstrate adequately. There are a number of things to plan for:

1. *Clarify the purpose.* It is important to decide exactly what
has to be demonstrated, and why. The demonstration should

concentrate upon the skill to be achieved, for it is not appropriate to include all aspects of related learning.

2. Be sure it is seen. The commonest reason for demonstrations not being seen is that they happen too quickly! It is important to avoid the temptation to give a slick performance. The object of the exercise is to assist the individual gain confidence that the skill will be mastered; a swift professional execution can often have exactly the opposite effect. The ideal speed for demonstration of injection technique, for instance, may be considerably slower than the usual speed of administration. Some things need to be seen in close-up and this will either limit the size of the group or necessitate the use of audio-visual material, such as film or larger than life models. Use of film or video has obvious benefits in providing close-ups. On the other hand, taking the object to be seen in close-up 'live' to group members singly or in parts has the additional advantage that they can touch the materials and ask questions immediately. In arranging close-ups it is important to get the perspective right: with a little thought it is usually possible to avoid presenting a mirror image.

3. Limit the distractions. Only essential items should be included in the demonstration itself. In teaching toothbrushing, for instance, the range of toothbrushes and pastes should be displayed separately; likewise in teaching stoma care, the range of appliances should be discussed before or after the technique of changing the bag is demonstrated. Having the full range of items which could be potentially relevant is a common source of distraction in demonstration. So too is the phenomenon of the missing item; everything necessary for the demonstration should be there from the beginning. Perhaps the commonest of all distractions is unnecessary or ill-timed commentary.

4. Organise the sequence. It is quite usual to organise a demonstration by showing the complete skilled performance initially and then examining component skills. Equally, it is possible to show individual difficult parts first, and then demonstrate the skilled performance. For instance, there may be an advantage in alerting learners to a wrist position or how a syringe is filled so that they may look out for these aspects when watching injection technique. People learn differently and it is more important to demonstrate what needs to be demonstrated than to progress through what appears to be a logical sequence.

5. *Prepare for repetition.* Parts of the demonstration which deal with vital or difficult aspects should be repeated. The nurse knows which aspects are vital and can plan for these. Identifying difficulties can only be done on an individual basis with the learner.

6. *Think through the details.* It is important to make provision for such items as electricity or water supply, waste disposal and protective clothing. For demonstrations to be useful all items of equipment should be to hand and in working order.

7. *Arrange follow-up.* The whole or parts of the demonstration may have to be repeated. Practice, initially with supervision, should be available to the learner soon after the demonstration.

Role play

Role play can be used to demonstrate opinions and feelings and to identify coping skills. Role playing makes use of drama technique in which learners act out and improvise roles which are assigned. Generally, the roles are improvised. For instance, in learning how to use communication techniques the parents of an adolescent, with whom they have been having difficulty talking, can role play with the teacher who can take the role of the adolescent. Subsequent analysis of the interaction is the valuable part of role playing.

To initiate a role play the scene should first be set. Then the actors' roles are described. Roles may be assigned or volunteers requested. Directions regarding the situation begin the role play. For instance, in the example given above, the teacher might say, 'I'll play the part of your adolescent son and we are discussing whether or not I can go out to a party on this school night.' Equally, it can be useful to ask the parent to play the part of the son, since it may be important for him to gain insight into his son's feelings.

After a short period of interaction, at a logical point, the role play should be stopped and analysis begun. Discussion of the interaction should come from all participants (including the audience if one is present) and learning may occur in several ways. In the instance of the parent/son role play:

1. The parents may identify why their adolescent son doesn't talk with them, or grows silent in discussions about his behaviour.
2. Suggestions about other ways to approach their son may be formulated when the identified communication patterns appear inadequate.
3. The parents may wish to learn other communication techniques to try with their son.
4. The parents may feel less frustrated and more willing to accept a changed level of communication (temporary or permanent) with their son.

Role play is equally applicable in affective learning. It has been included here under skills to emphasise that health teaching frequently deals with complex learning and that, in the acquisition of health-related skills, the learning is not merely psychomotor but also cognitive and often affective. Planning must take cognisance of this complexity.

CHOOSING TEACHING TECHNIQUES AND AIDS

Choice of technique

The choice of technique will be directed by the objectives the teacher and the learner wish to achieve. Other considerations in selection are: the number of participants, the type of material to be learned and the kind of learning to be promoted. There is no exact way of determining which teaching techniques will work. Much depends upon the personal styles of both learner and teacher.

Table 5.1 provides a quick reference to the variety of techniques, with indications of their use and a note of advantages and disadvantages.

Choice of aid

Appropriate use of teaching aids enriches the teaching and learning process. The stimulation of several senses helps to engage the learner more fully. It is beyond the scope of this text to deal in detail with the use of aids, but Table 5.2 provides a useful check list on a range of teaching aids which are readily available.

Table 5.1 Teaching techniques

What the health teacher hopes to accomplish	Kind of learning	Technique	Learner activity status	Advantages	Disadvantages	Example
1. Present information for consideration	Cognitive	— Lecture — Panel — Reading — Audiovisual aids eg. films, video	Passive	— Saves time and resources — Can teach a large number of learners — Learners feel secure in large group — Large amount of information can be presented	— Does not promote interaction or problem-solving — Teacher can't check individual progress — Same learning pace for all — Learner attentiveness low	Group of mothers of hydrocephalic babies to learn about condition and effects of shunt mechanism
2. Develop skills, psychomotor, interpersonal, etc.	Cognitive Psycho-motor Affective	— Demonstration and return demonstration — Simulation, — Role-playing	Active	*For 2 & 3 & 4* — Learner involvement — Permits interaction	*For 2 & 3 & 4* — High cost in time, resources — Socialization effects decrease concentration — Difficult to standardize learning situation for all learners	Learning to use crutches
3. Encourage understanding	Cognitive Affective	— Problem-solving exercises — Group participation	Active	— Facilitates evaluation by teacher — enables learner to risk in secure environment, to develop self-		Diabetic adolescent to understand and come to terms with her diabetes and to relate to others with diabetes

Objective	Domain	Active	Methods	Advantages	Disadvantages	Example
			— Guided project work — Programmed learning with feedback mechanism	confidence and interpersonal skills — develops problem-solving skills, self-evaluation — provides closer comparison with reality — With programmed learning—learner works at own pace: learning situation highly available	— With programmed learning — a lonely way to learn, may encourage a rigid view of correct responses—no opportunity to discuss	Young man to learn about possible consequences of his lifestyle which includes heavy drinking
4. Encourage examination of attitudes and values	Affective Cognitive	Active	— Group work-sharing experiences — counselling — games, role-playing — discussion, debate			

Table 5.2 Teaching aids (adapted from Hardy L K 1983, *Self-appraisal in health*. Scottish Health Education Group, p 13–14)

Aid	Advantages	Disadvantages	Example
1. Printed matter— books, handouts	— Allows self-pacing — Learners can refer to them when required — Reduces need for note-taking, therefore anxiety — Handouts can be made specific to individual learning needs — Supplements teaching session	— Books expensive and rapidly out of date — Handouts must be carefully planned and used appropriately. Should not replace teaching — Copyright law prohibits mass duplication of copyrighted material	In discussion of nutrition handouts about essential foodgroups and how to assess if family members are eating properly
2. Models of life, eg. skeleton	— Three dimensional — Resembles reality — Allows for close examination — Allows for practice — Visual and tactile senses stimulated	— May be expensive — Cannot replace reality — Use for small groups only	Use of doll in antenatal class demonstrations for expectant parents
3. Real specimens	— Present reality — Three dimensional — Visual and tactile senses stimulated	— Not easily available — Use for small groups only — May be expensive, difficult to store	Use of real baby in demonstrating baby bathing procedure
4. Graphics — charts, posters, drawings, photographs	— Visual sense stimulated — Promotes organisation and correlation of material — Helps to approximate reality — Easily stored, retrieved	— Production of materials should be of high standard — Use for small groups only	Used for discussion on alcohol problem in Western Europe as compared to British areas, eg. Scotland, England, Wales, Northern Ireland

	Advantages	Disadvantages	Uses/examples
5. Blackboard	— Visual sense stimulated — Inexpensive — Accommodates larger audience 30–50 — Allows for development of presentation — Allows for clarification, summary — Utilisable for a range of purposes	— Skill needed for effective use — If using during presentation, back to audience — Work erased	In sexuality teaching, use of this aid in diagramming orgasm response in males and females
6. Flannel board, magnetic board, bulletin board	— Easy to assemble and use — Can use repeatedly — Others may participate — Visual sense stimulated	— Limited use — Inappropriate for certain purposes and audiences	For young diabetics, choosing correct food items and creating a daily menu
7. Field trips	— Motivating — Active involvement — Presentation of reality	— Costly in time for organisation and accomplishment — Transport needed — For small appropriate groups only	For psychiatric patients, visits to shops to assess appropriate selection of clothing items
8. Overhead projection	— Visual sense stimulated — Easy to prepare and use — Available to large audiences — Can be preplanned or used on spot — Can illustrate process stages and develop material — Can allow for participation of learners	— Electricity required — Equipment costly — Transparencies need to be carefully planned for effective use	With renal failure patients, to explain the mechanism of kidney function and to illustrate what renal failure means

Aid	Advantages	Disadvantages	Example
9. Slides, film strips	— Available to large audiences — Can be adapted to self-learning programmes — Easy reproduction — Visual and auditory senses stimulated	— Need partial darkness for viewing — Colour slide duplication expensive — Needs careful presentation/slide order planning for effective use	For patients with recent colostomies, slide presentation of stoma appliance management
10. Films, video, television	— Resemble reality — Available to large audiences — Effective illumination of attitudes, values, can demonstrate skills — Visual and auditory senses stimulated	— Needs careful selection and previewing — Needs meaningful introduction and follow up discussion — Costly — Electricity required — All information in film may not be appropriate — No self-pacing — Person using must be proficient with equipment	With high school students, cases of drug dependency can be viewed and used as basis for discussion
11. Tape recordings	— Auditory sense stimulated — Self-pacing — Available to large audiences — Small recorders can be inexpensive, battery operated — Can be used for a variety of reasons	— Quality recordings may be difficult to obtain — Person using must be proficient with equipment	Tape initial session of a group in which health attitudes are discussed. Play back in later session to assess any changes
12. Expert contributors	— Presents reality — May provide a point of comparison — May command respect because of knowledge	— May not be easily available — May be expensive — May not be appropriate	Inviting an adolescent diabetic who is coping well to speak to a group of new juvenile diabetics about how he feels in relation to his condition

Guidelines for the selection of methods and aids

Teaching techniques and aids have to serve the purposes of both learner and teacher, as well as fitting the resources available. There are a number of questions to be considered in choosing a technique or aid:

1. Will it add to interest or understanding, or is it merely a distraction, or prop for the teacher?
2. How will it be acceptable to the learner?
3. Will it provide the opportunity for transfer of learning?
4. Will it involve the learner?
5. Is it appropriate to the learner's age, ability and experience?
6. Is it flexible?
7. Is it readily available?
8. Is it worth the cost?
9. Can the teacher use it with ease?
10. What contribution will it make to achieving the objectives for learning?

REFERENCES

Benne K D, Sheats P 1948 Functional roles and group members. Journal of Social Issues 4(2): 41–49

Bradshaw P W, Ley P, Kincey J A, Bradshaw J 1975 Recall of medical advice: comprehensibility and specificity. British Journal of Social and Clinical Psychology 14: 55–62

Levin K 1947 Frontiers in group dynamics. Human Relations 1: 5–42

Ley P 1973 A method for increasing patients' recall of information presented by doctors. Psychological Medicine 3: 217–220

Ley P 1976 Towards better doctor patient communications: contributions from social and experimental psychology. In: Bennett A E (ed) Communication between doctors and patients. Nuffield Provincial Hospitals Trust, Oxford University Press

Ley P, Spelman M S 1965 Communications in an out-patient setting. British Journal of Social and Clinical Psychology 4: 114–116

Ley P, Spelman M S 1967 Communicating with the patient. Staples Press, London

Pratt L, Seligman A, Reader G 1957 Physicians' views on the level of medical information among patients. The American Journal of Public Health 47: 1277

Riley C S 1966 Patients' understanding of doctors' instructions. Medical Care 4: 34–37

White R, Lippett R 1968 Leader behaviour and member reaction in three 'social climates'. In: Cartwright D, Zander A Group dynamics: research and theory, 3rd edn. Tavistock Publications, London

FURTHER READING

Abercrombie M L J 1970 Aims and techniques of group teaching. Society for
  Research into Higher Education, London
Cartwright D, Zander A 1963 Group dynamics: research and theory, 3rd
  edn. Tavistock Publications, London
Douglas T 1976 Groupwork practice. Tavistock Publications, London
McLeish J, Matheson W, Park J 1973 The psychology of the learning group.
  Hutchison University Library, London
Park M J 1973 The psychology of the learning group. Hutchison, London
Stephens M D, Roderick W (eds) 1971 Teaching techniques in adult
  education. David and Charles, London
Taylor L C 1971 Resources for learning. Penguin, Harmondsworth,
  Middlesex

Assessment and the
concept of need
Collecting information
Analysing information
Defining learning needs

6

Beginning the teaching-learning process: assessment of learning needs

OBJECTIVES

Study of this chapter will enable you to:

1. Discuss the concept of need.
2. Discuss the value of individualised assessment of needs.
3. Contrast the client's perception of needs with the nurse's as revealed by the review of research literature.
4. Discuss the nurse's role as advocate in respect of need.
5. Describe the process of analysing collected data.
6. Discuss the reasons for identifying specific learning needs.

ASSESSMENT AND THE CONCEPT OF NEED

The first phase in the teaching–learning process is assessment and its purpose is to determine what and how much the client needs, wants and is able to learn. The outcome of assessment will be the identification of needs for learning. These learning needs are identified by perceiving that a lack of learning has been or will be detrimental to the health status of the client. Thus, assessment data is analysed for *learning deficits* which guide the health teacher and learner in defining *learning needs.* Throughout this chapter it is assumed that identification of deficits is part of defining needs and will not be stated separately.

Professionals and patients may differ in their interpretation of what is necessary to learn and why. For this reason assessment has the best possible chance of success when the teacher and learner work together. Of course, there may have to be exceptions to this, such as when someone is too ill to take part or is unwilling or unable to accept responsibility. There are three aspects of the assessment process: collection of information, analysis of information and identification of learning needs (see Fig. 6.1).

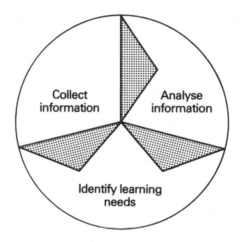

Figure 6.1 Assessment — systematic, continuous, productive

The three steps of assessment are interrelated and are not necessarily sequential, in the strict sense. Neither nurse nor client begins the assessment process with 'a blank sheet of paper'. The nurse has a mental framework based upon her experience of previous patients with similar needs. People usually have preconceptions of what is likely to be involved in certain illnesses and what may be expected of them. No one starts information-gathering for assessment without some idea of the type of analysis the data will be subjected to, and those assumptions about analysis are usually based upon having some insight into the kind of teaching objectives which are likely to be set.

A fundamental issue in assessment revolves around the concept of 'need'. Some definitions or statements about nursing discuss 'need' as if it were an absolute. This is not the case. 'Need' is a relative term. Not only are needs perceived differently by different people but also, they change over time.

Chambers and his colleagues (1980) have identified that the words want, need, demand, use and supply all may refer to the same thing or reflect different conceptual approaches depending on the orientation of the individuals considering them. Categorising needs helps to clarify what is meant and to alert the health teacher to differing views. Bradshaw (1972) has outlined four types of needs:

Normative needs. These are defined by the health care experts. They are not absolute but, instead, they reflect professional judgements. Value judgements may also play a role as professionals also have value sets of their own. For these reasons even the experts may disagree about aspects of need. Definitions of normative needs may conflict with the client's view of his own needs.

Felt needs. These needs equate with what the client wants. Demand for given services may be limited by the perceptions of an individual. In order to feel the need for a service, the health consumer has to be aware that it may be available. Though someone feels a need he may not be able to articulate it.

Expressed needs. These arise from felt needs, but are demonstrated in words or action. The client asks questions, forms a self-help group, or demands a service. Health teachers' assessments cannot rely only on expressed needs, for clients often will not ask or act.

Comparative needs. By studying similar populations it is possible to identify expressed needs and services which exist in one population but not the other. The observed difference prompts the deduction of need in the population under study. Frequently, this is a matter of expert opinion but not always. Also, the lack of service may not relate to need, depending on the reasons for introducing the service in the first place.

The difficulties associated with the definition of 'need' highlight the importance of client participation in assessment. Some needs are expressed freely and verbally. Other needs are not so readily verbalised. Many people find it difficult to say what they want and need to know about their health. Lack of familiarity with technical terms, embarrassment, feelings of social distance from health care professionals, denial of illness, pain and lack of privacy are just a few of the possible reasons for this. It is a common experience to be vague or to have mixed feelings about health-related information. Felt needs often exceed expressed needs.

An important part of collection of information for learning assessment is therefore concerned with ascertaining how nearly the expressed needs of a client reflect the felt needs. In assessing client perceived needs, the nurse has to be very ready to take into account what he has to say. Equally, it may be necessary to note what is not said or to determine whether what is said is what is meant. Clearly, the processes of data gathering and data analysis are interdependent.

Perception of need—the client's view

Research has found that, when asked about care, recently discharged hospital patients most frequently criticise the lack of information (Cartwright, 1964; Hugh Jones et al, 1964; Raphael, 1968). Poor explanations also proved dissatisfying to patients (Skipper et al, 1964) while medical language was considered a barrier to understanding (Linehan, 1966; Reynolds, 1978). Fear of pain and the unknown are frequently described concerns. In fact, Reynolds (1978) found people feared the unknown more than they feared the truth. Most people will therefore want information, but a few may not. Cartwright (1964) reported that 33% of the sample of 739 ex-hospital patients wanted to know 'as much as possible' about their disease. Only 10% of the same sample were consistently passive, not wanting much information nor asking questions. Benson et al (1977) found that patients wanted comprehensive information about intra-uterine devices. In contrast McIntosh (1976) discovered that the majority of subjects did not want to know more and described a situation in which lack of insight gave people hope. Such conflicting results reinforce the necessity for individual assessment.

Differences in desire for type as well as amount of information should be expected. Eardley et al (1975) found that people varied in the amount and type of advice they wanted. Needs have been found to change with social class (Beal & Dickson, 1974; Samson et al, 1971) and intelligence (Sims, 1977). Dodge (1969) described patients' information-seeking as 'survivalist'. The patients in her study attended to information they thought was important. In rank order the items were: dignosis, results of tests, aetiology of condition, future long-term effects and temporary activity restrictions. A number of other studies confirm that diagnosis is of primary concern to the individual patient (see reviews by Ley & Spelman, 1967; Hayward, 1975).

Perception of need—the nurses' view

Do nurses' perceptions of need differ from those of the client? Earlier it was suggested that they do. An example of this may be the case where the nurse assumes the client needs to know why his diet is restricted while he, on the other hand, may be interested only in what the restrictions are and how long they will be imposed. Equally, it could arise that the nurse assumes the patient requires to know only that pre-medication before surgery will cause drowsiness, while the patient feels entitled to know what the medication is called and how quickly it will take effect. Obviously, such differences in perception are unhelpful. They can and should be cleared by a few moments discussion.

On the other hand, some differences in perception of need may assist the process of assessment. The nurse has experience with other patients (normative information) and knowledge of research (comparative information) to draw on in identifying needs. This can be used to help patients identify or verbalise their needs.

Research has revealed something of how patients' and nurses' perceptions of need differ. Dodge (1972) found that patients valued information about long-term effects, how they would feel, how the illness was going to affect them, the degree of disability they would suffer, how lifestyles would be altered, their progress, diagnosis and prognosis, what was expected of them and how well they were coping with the condition. Contrary to these expectations, were the nurses' perceptions of need which included information on hospital routine and policy, timing of events, geography of the ward and relevant parts of the hospital, who's who on the staff, knowledge of investigations and treatment, what to expect during and after treatment, how they would feel after treatment and precautions and limitations associated with treatment. Different perceptions of need have been recorded by other investigators (Greene et al, 1980; Ashworth, 1978; Pratt et al, 1957).

Barriers to the perception of needs

A number of writers and researchers have addressed what inhibits clients' expression of needs. Linehan (1966) reported that patients were reluctant to ask nurses for information while Eardley et al (1975) found that morale and busyness of the ward affected patients' information-seeking.

Nurses may not respond well to clients' conversations and questions and thus may prevent further expression of needs. Faulkner (1980, 1981) discovered that nurses' conversation with patients was stereotyped and superficial and that they spent little time actually talking with patients. When student nurses were asked specific questions by patients they had difficulty in providing answers and seemed to have no clear idea of their role in giving information to patients. Melia (1981) referred to the student-nurse experience as 'nursing in the dark' as the students she interviewed told her that the ward staff did not give adequate information regarding the patient.

Redman (1971) and Pohl (1965) suggest a range of factors which interfere with nurses taking full responsibility for patient teaching: lack of information, inadequate preparation, belief that sharing knowledge with patients will decrease nursing power, lack of time, inadequate staffing, lack of nursing service support, poor communication between members of the health care team, lack of information-seeking by patients and perceived reluctance of doctors to allow nurses to teach. There is evidence (Carter, 1981; Webster, 1981; Marsh, 1979) that nurses lack relevant knowledge of teaching and have insufficient opportunity to practise teaching skills. Smith (1979) commented that a lack of commitment to health education may play a significant role. Wyness (1981) considered that conservative traditional views about the 'proper' role of the nurse may affect comprehensive assessment of needs.

Nurses may also have to change people's expectations of nurses as teachers if they are to help them articulate information needs. Cartwright (1964) found that 46% of patients expected doctors to be the main source of information while only 28% saw the ward sister providing information. Some barriers to accurate identification of needs are listed in Table 6.1.

Table 6.1 Barriers to identification of needs

Teacher Barriers to perception of client needs	*Learner* Barriers to expression of needs
— does not listen or respond to client questions — has insufficent information about client — lacks knowledge to deal with questions — discourages client participation to maintain control — lacks time due to poor ward organisation, or inadequate staffing — experiences little support from fellow professionals — lacks confidence — professional preparation has encouraged conservative beliefs about nurse's role in health teaching	— reluctance to ask questions — perceives ward too busy to seek attention — lacks language to request technical information — perceives professionals only as helpers, not teachers or informants — adopts passive role readily — not ready, nor motivated to participate — convinced by previous experiences that expression of needs is not welcomed — does not consider health teaching part of the nurse's role

The nurses' role as advocate in respect of need

In health care, needs appear to be limitless. Despite increases in the proportion of gross national product invested in health care (in 1983 Britain spent 6% on health care, the United States 10%), unmet needs continue to exist. With the economic recession of the 1970s and 1980s, health care systems in the Western world are having to ration resources available for health care. This is done in a variety of ways: by allowing waiting lists to grow; by increasing direct costs to the consumer; by limiting access by geographical region, age or clinical status, and so on.

The nurse's role in assessing needs is crucial and can be seen to encompass two aspects: firstly, she must assess, comprehensively, the needs of the individual(s) in her care, always conscious that his (or their) concept of need may differ from her own; and secondly, she must be capable of defining health education needs in general, in order to be able to make a case for resource allocation.

At a time when all industrialised societies are having to ration resources for health care, the nurse has a particularly important part to play, as consumer advocate, in establishing the case for the individual client's right to have adequate professionally provided health teaching.

COLLECTING INFORMATION

The main source of relevant data on current learning needs is the person who is to be taught. Secondary sources of information include the family, friends and significant others, the client's doctors, previous health records to which both nurses and doctors have contributed, social records, developmental records such as those kept by health visitors and family general practitioners, and results of X-rays and laboratory tests.

The simplest way to find out what someone needs to know is to ask him. Observation of his behavior may also provide information. Asking the patient about his health learning needs can be surprisingly easy. Sometimes it is enough just to arrange some privacy, set aside time, indicate interest and be prepared to listen. Often the first gathering of data related to health teaching needs will happen when the patient is interviewed as part of the overall assessment of nursing needs. Felt needs are more likely to be expressed if the patient feels at liberty to ask questions. The secret of success in the nursing assessment interview may lie in conveying to the patient or client that questions will be welcomed and answered if not by the interviewer then by another health care professional. It may also be helpful to indicate that other opportunities to ask questions are likely to occur and to suggest that the patient should jot down any questions which arise meantime.

What information should be sought? A number of complex forms for collecting data have been devised. There are arguments about whether such forms are useful, or whether they tend to prejudge the relevant issues. Wyness (1981) has offered the opinion that guides to assessment should be used, rather than detailed forms which may reduce individualised approaches.

As in any data-gathering session, general information must be recorded about the date of interview, the person's name, address, age, sex, religion, educational level and marital status. Figure 6.2 illustrates three areas in which further information might be obtained. At the beginning of the interview,

Patient's questions/comments
Anticipated needs (research based)
Diagnosis Treatment Investigations Prognosis Progress Self-care Routine
Aids/barriers to learning
Age Cognitive state Educational level Emotional level Grasp of technical   language Hearing Comfort Previous experience Sex Motivation to learn Attitude Learning ability

Figure 6.2 Areas for information seeking

or at least very early on, the client's questions and comments should be elicited. This will give insight into his perception of his needs and, as it introduces the session from the client's point of view, it may encourage continuing participation.

The way the person views his health situation should also be an area for assessment. For example, the questions below may help to discern his model of health:

> When you have been ill, what caused your illnesses?
> Could you have prevented any of the illnesses you've had?
> What do you do that helps you to feel well?
> What do you do that makes you feel unwell?
> Do you feel you are as healthy as you can be?

In some settings it may be appropriate for the nurse to perform a physical assessment to complement the data reported in the health history and to provide objective evidence of the person's health status. The nurse employs her senses of sight, hearing, touch and smell through the four techniques of inspection, palpation, percussion and auscultation (see Table 6.2 for definitions).

Table 6.2 The four techniques of physical assessment

1. Inspection	: to observe objectively, systematically, noting colour, odour and measurement as necessary.
2. Palpation	: to feel superficial and underlying structures of the body to note abnormalities.
3. Percussion	: to strike the surface of a body area with fingers to produce sounds that will indicate the character of underlying tissue.
4. Ausculation	: to listen to sounds produced by the heart, lungs, blood vessels, abdominal organs.

Recording the results of the health history and physical examination is important for later analysis and for communicating to other members of the health team. Recording expressed needs requires skill. It may be important, especially in an initial conversation, not to write down everything as it is said. Whenever possible it is advisable to give full attention to what is being said and to make arrangements for recording as soon afterwards as is feasible. Listing the patient's questions may be particularly useful. The number and type of questions may give clues as to the kind of information the patient wants and needs.

ANALYSING INFORMATION

Once initial information has been gathered, the analysis can begin. The purpose of analysis is to answer such questions as:

How willing and able to learn is this person?
How much does he need to know?
What is the nature of the learning task(s)?

Answers to these questions may be provided by utilising and building upon information gathered in the initial assessment. Many experienced nurses can quite quickly detail what a patient needs to know in given circumstances. The more experienced they are the more likely it is that they will also accurately determine how much he wants to know and is able to learn. Indeed, experienced nurses often collect and analyse information simultaneously so that in practice it seldom happens that the process by which such judgements are made is recorded. Consequently, there is little direct evidence to instruct practice at this time.

At its simplest, however, the analysis must deal with balancing three areas of concern. These are: items the patient says he needs to know about; items the nurse feels the patient may need to know despite his lack of expressed interest; and factors which are likely to affect his ability and willingness to learn.

Willingness and ability to learn are affected by a number of factors. Age or developmental level, sex, education level and experience, language and level of anxiety were discussed in Chapter 3. Knowledge of such factors helps the nurse anticipate some general areas of concern. Clearly, she may make some reasonably safe general assumptions about the different needs of a teenage female and an elderly man with the same diagnosis. What any particular person may need is a matter for more detailed consideration, however.

An obvious starting point for detailed individual analysis is with the list of questions asked by the patient at the initial assessment interview. Here again, the nurse must exercise judgement. Some questions clearly reveal considerable knowledge of diagnosis and a desire to get down to details. Others reveal ignorance or misinformation. But many questions cannot be interpreted at face value: pain, anxiety, first impressions of the health service, expectations and existing knowledge all affect what the individual may ask. Initial questions record what the person has been able to ask, not necessarily what he wants and needs to know.

Going back to the patient's original questions provides the nurse with a platform for a second and more analytical interview. It also serves to demonstrate to the patient that his questions matter to the nurse and that she is prepared to give him time to formulate further questions and seek the answers he wants.

The anticipated needs list prepared after the initial interview should also provide a framework for this second stage of assessment. The nurse will ask questions to ascertain how much the patient already knows about areas of importance she has identified. Often this can be done by general discussion of the areas concerned. In complex situations there may be value in using a check list or questionnaire.

As well as assessing learning needs and readiness to learn, it is necessary to consider the resources available for teaching. A main resource to consider is the nurse.

Yura & Walsh (1983) have documented the knowledge framework nurses need in order to assess patients' health needs as including knowledge of communication and helping relationships, human anatomy and physiology, chemistry, physics, microbiology, psychology, sociology, cultural anthropology, comparative religions, developmental psychology, mathematics, literature, art, philosophy, theology, psychopathology and pathophysiology. In addition the nurse, as health teacher, needs an up-to-date knowledge of health statistics, with particular reference to subgroups in the population. As well as having a sound scientific knowledge base, the nurse needs to have some knowledge of herself and be aware of how her value judgements, prejudices and previous experience of both illness and of health teaching may influence the resources she brings to bear upon any particular teaching session. For instance, repeated failure with a particular type of client — the alcoholic, the obese, the addicted cigarette smoker — may lead to undue pessimism; religious beliefs may make it difficult for the nurse to present options without bias in abortion counselling; unexplored feelings may block areas of discussion whilst counselling the bereaved.

Another important resource in health teaching, particularly

in clinical settings, is time. In analysing teaching needs, it is wise to consider realistically the time and personnel available for teaching. A teaching programme should be as comprehensive as possible, but there is no value in aiming at an all embracing programme if it cannot be accomplished.

Analysing the nature of the learning task

It is important to remember that most people who have something to learn about their health have an existing set of knowledge, beliefs and experience upon which to build. The learning task may therefore be concerned with unlearning or relearning. How the person enters the teaching–learning situation may be coloured by vicarious as well as actual experience, that is, he may have learned from others' stories of their contact with health care professionals. The person's attitudes towards these professionals should be elicited, for they may enhance or inhibit learning. Someone's experience with health care professionals may have convinced him that they never teach anything relevant. A negative previous encounter may make him reluctant to listen to any information offered by nurses. In such an instance it will clearly take time to establish a position of trust.

Sometimes, unlearning of roles may have to occur before other more specific learning needs can be focussed on. An example of this would be the woman who has had ulcerative colitis for years and in previous hospital experiences has tended to be a passive recipient of care. Exacerbation of the condition has resulted in the formation of an ileostomy and self-care has become an important teaching goal. Since she is accustomed to the nurse 'doing' all the care, she may have to learn a new role as an active participant.

Analysis of the learning task also involves considering the types of learning required and the challenges they present to the individual learner. In life, of course, the aspects of learning are interrelated. Nonetheless, some knowledge of the relative importance of each aspect may be helpful in selecting teaching methods, and so an attempt should be made to consider the relative weight of aspects of learning. For instance, is the learning mainly cognitive, or are there important affective elements which may dictate the time and setting required for learning?

It can be very difficult to weight the separate aspects of learning. What seem reasonable assumptions in very general terms may have little validity in particular instances. For example, it may seem reasonable to assume that the nature of disease or disability will dictate which aspects of learning gain precedence. Thus, cancer education may appear to be greatly concerned with emotional reactions and therefore affective learning. The individual cancer patient, however, may have already come to terms with the disease, perhaps through family experience, and may desire to concentrate upon acquiring information about the particular effects of current treatment. In the same vein, it might be assumed that people being prepared for surgery will require a cognitively based education programme, because of their obvious need for information, but any individual surgical patient may have considerable emotional barriers to learning.

Such examples illustrate the merits and limitations of the assumption that the nature of the disease or condition determines the nature of the learning task. Clearly, the characteristics of the individual are just as important as the nature of his illness. Relative weighting of factors is not as important as distinguishing the separate aspects of learning with respect to the challenges they pose to the individual.

A system of classifying types of learning in relation to teaching functions has been proposed (Bloom, 1956; Krathwohl et al, 1964). This suggests that there are levels of learning, and that they may be organised in a hierarchy of sophistication (see Chapter 3, Table 3.1). In some situations health teaching may be minimal, because the learning is simple. The preoperative patient who has to fast overnight, for instance, needs only to have the information and understand the rationale for it. The person with a stoma, on the other hand, has to be able to apply new knowledge and understanding in caring for his stoma and see relationships between stoma management and his lifestyle. In this case, the required learning is more complex.

Thus, in assessing the individual learner, certain questions can be posed: What type of learning is required, and at what level? Is the required cognitive learning concrete or abstract?

Are the needed motor skills beyond the manual dexterity of the patient at 7 years or 70? Is the necessary affective learning accomplishable in the short term, or should interim, and thus feasible, goals be set?

Most adults have a clear idea of how they learn, and so it may be possible to have the individual specify desired learning methods. It may also be helpful to ask the person how he usually learns things. What does he do when he has a number of things to memorise? How did he go about learning his hobby? With children, it may be necessary to involve parents in discussion about how learning may be accomplished. There can never be a formula, simple or complex, for predictable success in this area of assessment. Again, perhaps, the nature of the patient's questions and comments at initial interview and subsequently may give the best clues to the nature of the educational task.

In analysis, all available information about the person, from subjective and objective sources, is reviewed and processed. Knowledge, skills experience and sometimes intuition are used to interpret the data, and conclusions are drawn about the person's actual or potential learning needs. These are then validated with the patient or client (see Fig. 6.3).

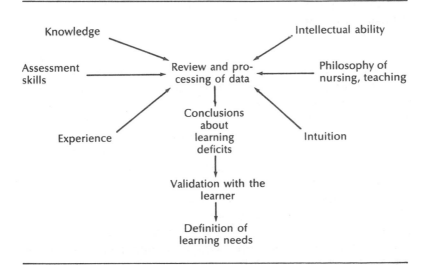

Figure 6.3 Factors involved in analysis

DEFINING LEARNING NEEDS

The assessment phase ends with the definition of the learning needs. In essence, the learning need is the statement which derives from the collection and interpretation of the data base and it is stated in a format which illustrates that an analytic approach helped to define it. For instance, a learning need might be stated:

> Mrs Smith needs to learn about stages of labour because she is seven months pregnant and is unable to describe or anticipate what she will experience when she begins her labour.

It would *not* be stated:

> Mrs Smith needs to learn about stages of labour because she fell down and broke her leg on Monday.

The second statement is clearly ridiculous. Listing learning needs helps to communicate to others the requirements for health teaching. The statements should be clear, simple, specific, concise and relevant to the nurse's role as health teacher. Occasionally, the learning needs identified are beyond the scope of the nurse, and should be referred to another health professional.

The list of learning needs implies a rank order of some kind. Usually, some needs require attention sooner than others. In the case of a severe diabetic, learning about insulin and its effects would be a first priority, while diet could come later since the client's meals are prepared in hospital. Before going home, nutritional information would become a critical need.

Redman (1975) has devised a system of priorising which is directly related to patient needs but it also assumes professional experience and judgement. She has described three categories: acute educational needs, when lack of understanding is causing physical danger or psychosocial anguish; preventive educational needs, which exist when individuals are threatened by conditions they lack the skills to handle; and, maintenance educational needs, which refer to needs of people who have to follow a medically prescribed regimen and may need frequent reteaching to maintain adequate levels of understanding and skill.

Maslow's hierarchy of needs may also provide a guide to assessing priorities. Maslow (1954) depicted human needs as falling into five categories. Starting with the most simple, *physiological needs* are basic to existence and include air, water, food, clothing and shelter; *safety needs* concern the need for survival; *social or affiliative needs* are those which incorporate significant relationships; *esteem needs* refer to those which enhance self-concept by achieving; and, *self-actualisation needs*, the highest level, involve the desire to achieve one's potential in life. When lower level needs are met, then needs at a higher level become prominent and require attention.

Use of Maslow's hierarchy of needs may be demonstrated in the case of the woman who has just been delivered of a

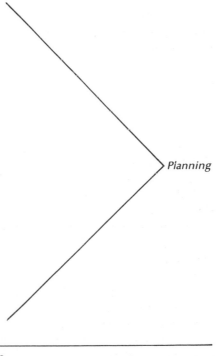

Assessment with the client:

1. Collect information

    – about the health learner from him; his health history and physical assessment; and other sources

    – about the health teacher whose level of learning facilitation depends on her knowledge, ability and attitude

2. Analyse the information

    – decide how willing and able the learner is

    – consider the nature of the learning tasks and decide upon the challenges they present to teacher and learner

3. Define the learning needs

    – refer to other teachers as necessary

    – priorise

Planning

Figure 6.4 The assessment process

normal healthy baby girl. Together, mother and nurse might list the learning needs and priorise them thus:

Learning need and rationale	Priority
Self-care and recognition of normal post-partum physiological changes because she is going home in 48 hours and will need to do self-assessment	1
Baby care to ensure survival and development of child	1
Contraception because this pregnancy was unplanned	2
Parenting skills because she and her partner are first time parents and have not attended parent-craft classes previously	2

Obviously the first two learning needs are immediately important for the survival of the mother and baby. The last two are important but can wait. Learning needs may thus be categorised as being short- or long-term. Figure 6.4 summarises the steps in assessment.

REFERENCES

Ashworth A P 1978 Communication in the intensive care unit. Nursing Mirror 146(7): 34–36
Beal J F, Dickson S 1974 Social differences in dental attitude and behaviour in West Midland mothers. Public Health 89(1): 19–30
Benson H, Gordon L, Mitchell C 1977 Patient education and intra-uterine contraception: a study of two package inserts. American Journal of Public Health 67(5): 446–449
Bloom B S (ed) 1956 Taxonomy of educational objectives, handbook 1: cognitive domain. David McKay Company, New York
Bradshaw J 1972 A taxonomy of social needs. In: McLachlan G (ed) Problems and progress in medical care. Essays on Current Research 7th Series, Nuffield Provincial Hospitals Trust, Oxford University Press, London
Carter E 1981 Ready for home? Nursing Times 77(19): 826–829
Cartwright A 1964 Human relations and hospital care. Routledge & Kegan Paul, London
Chambers L W, Woodward C A, Dok C 1980 Guide to health needs assessment: a critique of available sources of health and health care information. Department of Clinical Epidemiology and Biostatistics, McMaster University, Hamilton, Ontario

Dodge J S 1969 Factors related to patients' perceptions of their cognitive needs. Nursing Research 18(6): 502–513

Dodge J S 1972 What patients should be told: patients' and nurses'beliefs. American Journal of Nursing 72(10): 1852–1854

Eardley A, Davis F, Wakefield J 1975 Health education by chance: the unmet needs of patients in hospital and after. International Journal of Health Education 18(1): 19–25

Faulkner A 1980 Communication and the nurse. Nursing Times 76(21) Occasional paper: 93–95

Faulkner A 1981 Aye there's the rub. Nursing Times 77(8): 332–336

Greene J Y, Weinberger M, and Mamlin J J 1980 Patient attitude towards health care: expectation of primary care in a clinical setting. Social Service and Medicine Oxford 14a(2): 133–138

Hayward J 1975 Information: a prescription against pain. Royal College of Nursing, London

Hugh-Jones P, Tansor A R, Whitby C 1964 Patients' view of admission to a London teaching hospital. British Medical Journal 2(5410): 661–664

Krathwohl D K, Bloom B S, Masia B B 1964 Taxonomy of educational objectives, handbook 11: affective domain. David McKay Company, New York

Levin L S 1973 Patient education and self-care: how do they differ Nursing Outlook March: 170–175

Ley P, Spelman M S 1967 Communicating with the patient. Staples Press, London

Linehan D T 1966 What does the patient want to know? American Journal of Nursing 66(5): 1066–1070

Marsh N 1979 The patient needs to talk. Nursing Mirror 148(26): 16–18

Maslow A 1954 Motivation and personality. Harper and Row, New York

McIntosh J 1976 Patients' awareness and desire for information about diagnosed but undisclosed malignant disease. The Lancet ii: 300–303

Melia K 1981 Student nurses' accounts of their work and training: a qualitative analysis. Unpublished Doctoral dissertation, University of Edinburgh

Pohl M L 1965 Teaching activities of the nursing practitioner. Nursing Research 14(1): 4–11

Pratt L, Seligmann A, Reader G 1957 Physicians' view on the level of medical information among patients. American Journal of Public Health 47(10): 1277–1283

Raphael W 1969 Patients and their hospitals. King Edward's Hospital Fund, London

Redman B K 1971 Patient education as a function of nursing practice. Nursing Clinics of North America 6: 573–580

Redman B K 1975 Guidelines for quality of care in patient education. Canadian Nurse 71: 19–21

Reynolds M 1978 No news is bad news: patients' views about communication in hospital. British Medical Journal 1 (6128): 1674–1676

Samson C D, Wakefield J, Pinnock K M 1971 Choice or chance? How women come to have a cytotest done by the family doctor. International Journal of Health Education 14(2): 127–138

Sims P 1977 The dental habits dental knowledge and dental attitudes of Southend teenagers 1975. Public Health 91(4): 189–201

Skipper J K, Tagliacozzo D L, Mauksch H O 1964 What communication means to patients. American Journal of Nursing 64(4): 101–103

Smith J P 1979 The challenge of health education for nurses in the 1980s. Journal of Advanced Nursing 4: 531–543

Webster M E 1981 Communication with dying patients. Nursing Times 77(23): 999–1002

Wyness M A 1981 Assessment: one element of patient education. In: Health teaching: A nursing activity, Scottish Health Education Group, Edinburgh

Yura H, Walsh M 1983 The nursing process, 4th edn. Appleton-Century Crofts, Norwalk, Connecticut

FURTHER READING

Dubrey Sister R J 1982 Promoting wellness in nursing practice. C V Mosby Company, London

Lamonica E L 1979 The nursing process: a humanistic approach. Addison-Wesley Publishing Company, London

Narrow B W 1979 Patient teaching in nursing practice: a patient and family centered approach. John Wiley & Sons, New York

Redman B K (ed) 1981 Issues and concepts in patient education. Appleton-Century-Crofts, New York

Planning
Who plans?
The mechanics of
  planning
The teaching plan

7

Planning: preparation for teaching

OBJECTIVES

Study of this chapter will enable you to:

1. Describe the nature of planning as it applies within the teaching process.
2. Discuss why learner participation is crucial in planning.
3. State the purposes of using objectives.
4. Identify instructional objectives which are stated in behavioural terms.
5. Write instructional objectives which indicate how teaching may be evaluated.
6. Discuss the benefits and limitations of written objectives as planning tools for teaching.
7. Discuss the advantages and limitations of written teaching plans in health teaching.
8. Draw up a teaching plan in outline form in relation to specified objectives.
9. Draw up a teaching plan in outline form suited to the needs of a specified individual.

PLANNING

It is not unusual for people to say they have a plan when what they really mean is that they know what they usually do in given circumstances. In other words, what passes for planned action may be no more than observance of routine. In health teaching it is important that planning is an active process, involving the identification of alternative ways to meet specified goals and decisions about the best way to achieve desired results. Planning should also involve the identification of possible pitfalls, and preparation for avoidance. The prudent teacher will have plan B ready in case plan A fails. Planning is about thinking things through: it requires imagination and lateral, as well as logical, thinking. A plan is more a state of mind than a piece of paper.

Planning, therefore, is a process which directs the health teacher and health learner toward certain actions which will facilitate learning.

WHO PLANS?

The person to be taught, and his relatives, should be involved in planning for health teaching, as well as the relevant health care professionals. Doctors and nurses have separate, though complementary, roles to play. In patient education the doctor may, in some circumstances, be required to indicate a willingness to have teaching carried out. Redman (1980) indicates that this is usual practice in parts of the United States of America, and that written teaching plans may include a space where the doctor's permission for teaching is recorded.

In the British Isles the arrangement is usually unwritten, literally and metaphorically, in as much as the differences in medical and nursing roles in health education are not usually spelt out and may depend largely upon custom and usage, or 'tradition'. The doctor may also expect, or be expected, to assess the person's information needs in relation to such aspects as diagnosis, investigations and treatment, and he will usually assume responsibility for communicating most if not all of this information to the person. The nurse completes the process of assessing needs, often paying particular attention to affective and psychomotor needs. She will be concerned to weigh the person's needs with his ability and willingness to learn, and her planning activity may be related to determining how the doctor's instructions about information to be communicated may be interpreted in the individual's best interest.

The client's participation in planning is encouraged to the extent possible for him. Most critically ill people will not have the desire to be involved. Still, even in these cases, the nurse has a responsibility to convey to the client or his family what she has planned and why. This allows for a degree of participation and control on the part of the ill person. The professional health teacher's ultimate goal is that the client become self-motivated and self-caring about his health; thus, the planning phase in teaching should address short-term and long-term goals in which the nurse's role is seen to decrease as a result of goal achievement. Figure 7.1 illustrates how this

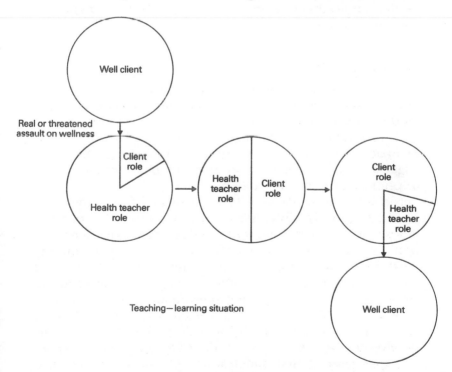

Figure 7.1 Progression of client and health teacher roles (adapted from Ewing, 1984)

can happen. The client role can be defined more broadly in the case of the severely ill or comatose person to include the family or significant others. It is precisely these people who, with some knowledge of the individual, can describe the type of person he is, what he likes or doesn't like and so on. Their role, like the nurse's, must decrease as he becomes more able to participate.

THE MECHANICS OF PLANNING

The planning process involves checking the priorising done at the end of the assessment phase; setting learning objectives; and, deciding on the teaching which will achieve the objectives by considering methods and learning aids, the environment and the teacher's capabilities. Lastly, the client's motivation level and readiness to learn have to be evaluated and encouraged.

Learning priorities

In the assessment phase, learning priorities are established by deciding which items are most important and have to be attended to first.

Categorisations like Maslow's (1954) hierarchy of needs or Redman's (1975) guidelines, are useful tools for priorising as suggested in Chapter 6. In the planning phase other aspects of priorising can be considered.

The learning needs have to be separated from other care needs. Obviously, only essential nursing can be carried out in a situation which is life threatening or demands speedy action. For a person suffering from acute bronchitis the priority must be to relieve breathlessness. Subsequently, however, it may be appropriate to include teaching aimed at reducing smoking as one part of nursing intervention. In less acute situations, the challenge is to identify the sequence of lessons most likely to be useful to the individual. Should explanations be given before new skills are tried? Or will there be benefit in experimenting first and learning the details later? Such questions can only be answered in the light of individual circumstances and there is no sure formula for getting it right.

In patient education within hospital, it may be necessary to identify short-and long-term goals for health teaching and to concentrate within the period of hospitalisation upon short-term goals. The nurse then has to decide in which areas health teaching is most needed. Again, this must be considered in conjunction with the client for he will be able to verbalise his personal view of which long-term goals he is capable of achieving outside of hospital.

Setting objectives

Specifying objectives is a necessary part of planning to teach. The process of writing objectives helps to clarify purpose, establish what content is relevant and realistic, and identify suitable teaching methods. Additionally, if objectives are well written they provide a means to evaluate teaching. Clarifying the purpose of teaching and establishing what content will be relevant are often the most difficult parts of the teaching process. In any health lesson there will be a small central core of knowledge and skills which is essential for the individual to master. Beyond that are many areas which may or may not need to be included in order to help the individual understand the information or develop the skills he needs to have. The extent and nature of that extra material varies, as some people need more help to understand things than others, and the background knowledge and experience individuals bring to the learning situation is of almost infinite variety. Beyond the range of things needed to aid understanding are the many items of interest which could be included in a teaching session. Adding items of interest is an important part of planning for teaching because it may motivate the learner if his interest is captured. There is always the temptation, however, to add the interest items in response to the teacher's need for stimulation as much as to learner needs. Writing objectives for teaching helps to clarify whose needs are being met by the teaching plan.

In everyday use, the words 'aim' and 'objective' are interchangeable. When applied to educational planning, however, the term 'objective' takes on a particular meaning: educationalists use it to connote a carefully worded statement which precisely identifies the intention of the teacher. In order to

emphasise that the term has precise meaning, some educationalists apply the adjectives 'instructional' or 'behavioural'
to objectives. Mager (1962) described three main characteristics of a usefully stated behavioural objective:

1. It is stated in learner terms.
2. It describes terminal behaviour.
3. It has inbuilt evaluation.

1. Stating objectives in terms of the learner

An objective should state what the teaching is intended to
accomplish. Some teachers assume this means writing down
what the teacher will do. However, since learning is also an
active part of the teaching–learning process it is equally possible to write down what the learner will be expected to do as
a result of teaching. Writing an objective in learner, rather than
teacher, terms provides an instant challenge in terms of evaluation of the lesson. Consider the example below:

Objective A	*Objective B*
The teacher will out-line the role of sugar in the formation of dental caries.	The learner will be able to describe the role of sugar in the formation of dental caries.

Objective A may be met if the teacher merely talks for an
allotted time. There is no way to be sure objective B has been
met without testing the learner in some way.

So the first rule in writing objectives is to express them in
terms of the learner, showing what he will be able to do as
a result of a lesson or lessons.

2. Describing the learner's terminal behaviour

In the example above there is a statement about the learner's
terminal behaviour, in other words, what he will be able to
do after teaching. In this case, he will be able to describe
something. Useful description of terminal behaviour largely
depends upon using the right verb. In the example given, the
word 'describe' was used, which means that the objective, as
stated, specified action which is capable of being observed.
Some verbs specify action which is not directly observable.
Again, contrast the two objectives stated below:

Objective A
The learner will know about the role of sugar in the formation of dental caries.

Objective B
The learner will be able to describe the role of sugar in the formation of dental caries.

It is impossible to observe 'knowing'. The learner will have to be asked to do something additional to demonstrate his knowledge. Describing can be observed, however, so 'describe' is a better verb than 'know' to use in defining the terminal behaviour. So the second rule when writing objectives is to choose language which determines learner actions that are capable of direct observation.

3. Building in evaluation

An objective should be stated in terms of observable learner behaviour. Additionally, the objective should be capable of evaluation, and this means that somewhere within the objective there should be an indication of the standard which will be used to judge the learner's performance. In the example given above, the person is expected to be able to describe the role of sugar in the formation of dental caries, but there is no indication of how detailed or accurate the description needs to be. As it stands, the objective does not specify this, and so it is a less useful statement of educational intent than it might be. A third rule in writing objectives, then, is to ensure that each objective identifies the criteria required for successful performance of the terminal behaviour.

In the instance examined above, if a fairly simple description of the role of sugar is all that is required, then it would be easy to specify the nature and standard of performance required of the learner by indicating, separately, the items which should be mentioned. So that the objectives might be written thus:

Objective
As a result of teaching, the learner will be able to describe the role of sugar in the formation of dental caries; i.e.
1. Sugar is metabolised by bacteria in plaque, with resultant formation of acid. The acid attacks the tooth enamel and caries result.
2. Increased sugar consumption increases the rate of formation of plaque.

For most health teaching this is likely to be a satisfactory way of identifying evaluation criteria. Sometimes, however, more detailed knowledge is required, perhaps because the person has to grasp an understanding of a complex disease process or because the particular person concerned is especially curious about details and causation. In such an instance, the single global objective may have to be replaced by a more detailed series of objectives, distinguished in relation to the cognitive, affective and psychomotor learning required. In the dental health example outlined earlier, there are cognitive and affective learning objectives which might be written thus:

Objectives	Level of achievement
After teaching the health learner will:	
Cognitive learning	
1. identify sucrose as the sugar most implicated in dental caries;	1. knowledge
2. describe the composition of plaque;	2. knowledge
3. recount at least one experiment demonstrating the production of acid after sugar ingestion;	3. knowledge
4. identify patterns of sugar ingestion most likely to contribute to the development of caries;	4. application
5. name 3 foods with high and 3 foods with low sucrose content.	5. comprehension
Affective learning	
1. hold the attitude that avoiding dental caries is worth the self-denial involved in sugar regulation;	1. valuing

Objectives	Level of achievement
2. believe that dental caries is preventable;	2. valuing
3. believe that preventing dental caries is desirable;	3. valuing
4. believe that personal efforts will make an impact on the prevention of dental caries;	4. valuing
5. regulate sugar intake so as to minimise acid attack on tooth enamel.	5. characterisation

Writing separate objectives for cognitive, affective and psychomotor learning completes the analysis of the educational task. Note that there has been an assumption made about the attitude that for sugar regulation to be worthwhile, the attitude will have to be supported by a cluster of beliefs about the benefits and probability of prevention. Also, by specifying what level of achievement is desired in each learning domain, it can be seen that the affective learning desired requires the highest level of learning. Such detailed analysis of objectives raises questions about the reactions and learning capabilities of the individual, and it becomes obvious that it will be essential to involve the person himself in the analysis and planning tasks. Objectives for sugar regulation, for instance, can only be set realistically in the light of what the individual contracts to do. Ideally, sweet things between meals should be avoided completely and there should be a move from highly refined sugar in the diet to other sugars and sweeteners. For some people this will require only minimal adjustment. Others may opt to begin by cutting out sweets between meals or by contracting to reduce sweet consumption while watching television. This example illustrates the danger of pressing on regardless, in pursuit of well written objectives. Though there are rules to follow, they should be applied to aid the thinking processes surrounding the planning of teaching, rather than blindly followed.

Writing objectives can be difficult, but the benefits are that the purpose of teaching may become clarified, and the means of evaluation identified. If teacher and learner alike have a clear idea of what is to be accomplished then it will be possible to assess what is being achieved. One way to clarify purpose is to try to be as unambiguous as possible in stating the standard of performance which will be required of the learner.

Limitations of behavioural objectives

The use of behavioural objectives is sometimes criticised, on the grounds that they may lead to inflexibility in teaching. Another criticism is that by concentrating upon what is measurable, they limit the view of what it is possible to teach. These potential dangers are particularly likely to be damaging in health teaching, since involving the learner necessitates a flexible and wide approach. Nonetheless, the benefits of attempts to clarify teaching purpose are obvious and, on balance, it is likely that the advantages of well written objectives will outweigh the disadvantages, so long as objectives are used as an analytic tool in the planning process and not as an end in themselves.

Preparing to teach—methods, aids, environment, health teacher and health learner

When learning objectives have been formulated, the participants to the teaching–learning process decide on the methods, aids and environmental requirements which will enable those objectives to become operational. The information provided in Chapters 3 and 4 help in this decision making. At this point general comments only are made concerning these aspects.

Choosing a method of teaching

If objectives are specified in cognitive, affective and psychomotor terms this helps to clarify the type of teaching needed. Consider the cognitive and affective objectives in the dental health example quoted earlier. The cognitive objectives may

be met by some didactic teaching: a leaflet might do, provided it is at the right reading level, and assuming that the
person has no undue suspicion of scientific evidence. The
affective objectives present a very different challenge. Here
the learner needs to have a chance to explore beliefs and test
them with others. Less didactic teaching is needed. The person will either have to have a chance to challenge the nurse's
position on self-denial of sugar or, ideally, be helped to examine the issue with a group of others.

Choosing aids to enhance learning

A learning aid is supposed to facilitate learning in some way,
not take up time or give the health educator something with
which to 'jazz-up' the teaching session. The aid should amplify
rather than duplicate any factual information. If it introduces
unnecessary extra material which is likely to confuse it
should be abandoned.

If audio-visual aids are to be used it is important to check
that machinery will operate as anticipated. The only way to do
this is to rehearse its use: make sure slides are in sequence,
and that they project the right way up, ascertain the position
of electrical points, check on whether an extension cord is
needed, adjust the position of the screen . . . the list is end-
less. These preparations should be done in advance, as it may
cause irritation or even anxiety if visual apparatus has to be
adjusted as the teaching begins. It is less amusing than generally supposed to give the lame excuse that technology always fails.

Planning the teaching environment

Some aspects of the teaching environment may be difficult to
control: a ward can be noisy, for instance, and there may be
a lack of privacy. It is important to do whatever possible to
manipulate such factors. There may be a side-ward or day-
room available, or perhaps it would help to screen the bed.
It goes without saying that it will help to have the opportunity
to sit down comfortably in relaxed surroundings when very
personal concerns are under discussion.

As important as the physical setting is the psychological setting. It is important to have the person feel confident that the teacher intends to communicate clearly and will give undivided attention to the learner. In group settings it may be useful to arrange furniture so that people can see each other. In some situations a cup of tea or coffee may ease the initial moments and give groups of relative strangers the opportunity to relax before the session begins.

Planning for teacher involvement

Some kinds of teaching are more demanding than others. If attitudes and beliefs are to be examined the nurse may need to consider her own before the lesson. If feelings are to be explored it is as well to consider possible personal reactions and the extent to which it will be, both personally and professionally, acceptable and possible to share feelings with someone else with whom there may be established role expectations as client or patient. The planned teaching should not exceed the capabilities nor go against the usual inclinations of the teacher concerned. Table 7.1 illustrates a useful self-check list. Where there is a potential problem of values-conflict it may be wiser for another nurse to take over teaching in a given area or with a particular person.

Table 7.1 Self-exploration checklist for use in planning teaching

What are my values and attitudes related to this aspect of health/health care?

How do I feel about interacting with this person? Can I respect him? Will I be able to accept his views? Do I intend to act as informant, teacher, persuader or enabler?

Are there differences of language, age and social class? Can anything be done about them?

Is what I do congruent with what I prescribe? Need it be congruent?

Planning for client involvement

The motivation level and state of readiness of the client will have been assessed and will have an impact on planning. The client who has just had a myocardial infarction may be well motivated to learn how to avoid further cardiac incidents by reducing the stress he has been experiencing, stopping smoking and maintaining his weight at an appropriate level. However, his readiness to learn may initially be complicated by factors such as fear and pain. Thus, the health teacher plans the teaching sessions keeping these factors in mind.

In some cases a reluctance to learn may be overcome by encouraging a commitment of some sort. Contracts can be verbal or written. Contracts need to be reviewed regularly to assess progress, to change objectives if necessary as more data collection occurs and to remind both participants of their commitment. In some situations it may be easier to carry out these tasks with written contracts, and if this is so the client or patient should always have a copy of his own to review.

It is also, at this point in planning, wise to reflect on the information gathered about the client's past learning experiences and the ways in which, reported by him, he learns best. The learner who has always had difficulty with concept learning when teachers 'talk' through the ideas will need a different approach.

THE TEACHING PLAN

Teaching plans are not always written down. A mental checklist and plan of action may be all that is needed in some instances, and has the advantage of saving time in documentation. It is certainly more important to make a plan than to be in possession of a written sheet purporting to be a plan. Nonetheless, written plans are useful, especially in complex teaching, since the very act of writing the plan may trigger further analysis and planning. Written plans also provide reminders for action, a framework for documentation and evaluation of teaching, and serve as a communication device to other involved professionals.

Written teaching plans will vary, but any teaching plan should have some key elements:

— a description of the learner(s)
— a list of learning needs priorised
— a statement of objectives
— a note of aids and barriers to learning
— an outline of content

— an indication of sequence
— a description of teaching method
— notes on the use of teaching aids
— notes on environmental preparation
— actual outcome (evaluation notes)

Teaching plans may be problematic in that they may be poorly utilised. They must be written in clear concise language so that fellow health teachers readily comprehend their intent. Strict adherence to a plan may reduce flexibility with changing needs. Use of a plan, therefore, should encourage constant re-assessment of needs, priorities and teaching actions. By having two copies of the plan with two people reviewing it and referring to it, both the health learner and teacher measure progress and can be accountable.

Example of a teaching plan

In the case below only parts of the plan are fully developed. It is acknowledged that clients, newly diagnosed as having diabetes mellitus, would have a number of other learning needs which are not presented here.

Date:	26 March 1984
Name:	Ann Smith *Age:* 18
Address:	University residence
Marital Status:	Single
Occupation:	1st year university student, studying philosophy
Religion:	non-practising
Next of kin:	mother Mrs J Smith
Address:	City, 200 miles away
Diagnosis:	Diabetes mellitus, is aware of diagnosis
Previous medical history:	reports 'I've never been sick before except for the odd cold'

Learning needs	*Priority*
1. to develop self-care knowledge and skills to prevent complications and optimise health;	Short term

2. to accept that regulation of blood sugar   Longer term
   will have to become a conscious aspect
   of lifestyle.

Aids or barriers to learning

Quick to grasp detail. Appears confident.

Environmental concerns

Prefers one to one sessions with privacy.

Teaching plan

Learning need	Objectives—with learning the client will:	Teaching action (Methods & Aids)
1. to develop self-care skills to prevent complications and optimise health	1. describe the patho-physiology of diabetes — cause — complications — treatment	Booklets × 2, discussion
	2. correctly test urine —relate results to status of diabetes	Explanation, demonstration, return demonstration, supervised practice
	3. choose correct insulin — drug name — action	Work with vials, drug information
	4. correctly calculate insulin dosage — relate to acidosis and hypoglycaemia	Explanation, supervised practice

Learning need	Objectives — with learning the client will:	Teaching action (Methods & Aids)
	5. safely administer injections — correct technique — review aspects of safety	Explanation, demonstration, return demonstration, supervised practice
	6. discuss the relationship of diet to diabetes — choose appropriate foods and explain their relevance	Refer to dietician, use menu sheets
	7. discuss the relationship of exercise to diabetes	Booklets, discussion, use case examples
	8. explain reasons for special care: of feet, eyes, skin, minor illnesses	Booklets

Need and objective	Dates of teaching	Evaluation date	Notes (initialled)
1:1	26/3/85	26/3/85	— Appeared eager to learn. Asked questions — Would like more than booklets. One of British Diabetic

Need and objective	Dates of teaching	Evaluation date	Notes (initialled)
	28/3/85	29/3/85	Association suggested books given. (LC) — Seems to feel overwhelmed by all the facts on diabetes. Is able to correctly identify cause and complications of condition but is having difficulty relating how the treatment works.
	28/3/85	2/4/85	Introduced to another client with diabetes who felt same way when first learning. (LKH) Is proud to be able to explain disease process. Says 'Mary (fellow patient) told me that I would be learning all my life about diabetes and all that I learned would help me to feel well.' (LKH)

In diabetic education it is important to realise that the hospital nurse can only begin a process which will continue throughout the rest of the person's life. In evaluation it is therefore important to distinguish short-and long-term goals. The immediate concerns are whether the patient is learning the things it is appropriate to learn at this stage and whether the teaching is being done in the most helpful way. Ascertaining that does not have to depend upon an evaluation form or research technique. Perhaps the best way to find out is to ask the patient!

Once planning has concluded, action is taken (see Fig. 7.2 for continuous nature of the teaching–learning process) and teaching occurs.

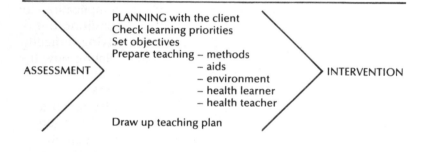

ASSESSMENT

PLANNING with the client
Check learning priorities
Set objectives
Prepare teaching – methods
　　　　　　　　 – aids
　　　　　　　　 – environment
　　　　　　　　 – health learner
　　　　　　　　 – health teacher
Draw up teaching plan

INTERVENTION

Figure 7.2　The planning process

REFERENCES

Ewing G 1984 A study of the post-operative nursing care of stoma patients during appliance changes. Unpublished doctoral dissertation, University of Edinburgh.
Mager R F 1972 Preparing instructional objectives. Fearon Publishers, Palo Alto, California
Maslow A 1954 Motivation and personality. Harper and Row, New York
Redman B K 1975 Guidelines for quality of care in patient education. Canadian Nurse 71: 19–21
Redman B K 1980 The process of patient teaching in nursing, 4th edn. C V Mosby, St Louis

FURTHER READING

Billie D A 1981 Practical approaches to patient teaching. Little, Brown and Company, Boston

Lamonica E L 1979 The nursing process: a humanistic approach. Addison-Wesley Publishing Company, London
Mager R F 1972 Goal analysis. Lear Siegler Inc/Fearon Publishers, Belmont, California
Murray R B, Zentner J P, 1979 Nursing concepts for health promotion, 2nd edn. Prentice-Hall, Englewood Cliffs, New Jersey
Wilson-Barnett J (ed) 1983 Patient teaching. Churchill Livingstone, Edinburgh
Zander K S (ed) 1978 Practical manual for patient teaching. C V Mosby, St Louis

8

Implementation of teaching plans

OBJECTIVES

Study of this chapter will enable you to:

1. Utilise the ideas and theories presented in earlier chapters in implementing health teaching.
2. Demonstrate, by developing your own case study, the ways in which the assessment and planning phases relate to the process of implementation.

The implementation phase of the teaching–learning process activates all of the joint plans made by the health teacher and the learner. It is in the act of teaching that the accuracy and depth of assessment are tested and plans are validated, and careful preparations leading to health teaching are proven to be effective or ineffective.

The aim of health teaching is the achievement of the objectives which were defined in the planning stage. While the teaching plan is being carried out, ongoing assessment and planning continues, as the nurse remains alert to new facts about the client. These new facts and on-going evaluation about the outcome of teaching may create changes in the teaching plan.

It is in the implementation phase that the nurse uses her theory base and skills actively, creatively and intelligently to help the client to learn about his health behaviour. This phase is the most demanding for the health teacher, who has to interact intentionally and effectively.

In this chapter, examples are presented to illustrate the process which occurs in health teaching. Each has a dynamic development which acknowledges that phases of the teaching–learning process are continuous and interactive. None represents an actual situation, but each has been chosen to reflect recent experiences in health teaching.

EXAMPLE 1: STOMA APPLIANCE MANAGEMENT

Assessment

Personal data   *Date*: 27 March 1985
Name: Mr Jack Royal
Address: 121 Rue Road,   *Telephone*: 666 1101
       Edinburgh
D.O.B.: 21 October 1948   *Occupation*: High School
                                  teacher   of
                                  Science
Marital Status: Married, 2   *Religion*: non-practising
                 children
                 ages 4 and
                 6
Height: 190.5 cm   *Weight*: 79.5 kg
Reason for contact: Client has a newly formed colostomy and is needing help learning to care for it.
Diagnosis: Cancer of the rectum. Transverse colostomy performed 26 March 1985. Client was an emergency admission. No pre-operative counselling or teaching was accomplished.

Physical assessment

Mr Royal is one day post operation. He is a clean looking, well-proportioned individual who appears to be in no distress. He looks his stated age of 36 years. He is sitting up in bed speaking to his wife as I approach. He has an intravenous line running into a brachial site on his left arm. He is located in a ward bed.

Vital signs:

Temperature: oral, 8 minute reading 37.2° centigrade

Pulse: right radial site, 86 per minute, regular

Respiration: 26 per minute, regular

Blood pressure: right brachial site, client sitting up in bed, reading 144 (systolic)/76 (diastolic—last sound heard).

Physicians' notes on physical assessment reveal that Mr Royal has been experiencing lower abdominal pain for some time but thought it was due to occupational stress. Other than the abdominal symptoms, he reported no problems and a physical examination revealed no other health deficits.

He was admitted with acute lower abdominal pain experienced over a 24-hour period. Surgery was an immediate indication.

Psychosocial assessment

Mr Royal is a married 36 year-old secondary school teacher with two young children. He has been working as a teacher for 13 years but has been at his present school for only 2 years, as principal teacher in the science department. He says that: 'The job has been tough. There's a lot of responsibility and the school has a reputation for science teaching the headmaster would like to maintain.' Mrs Royal reports that her husband's personality has changed since he took on the principal teacher position: 'He used to be easy-going, played with the children (4-year-old son, 6-year-old daughter) and planned outings with me. Now he never seems to be home and when he is he works.'

Mrs Royal works part-time as a nurse at a nursing home. She enjoys this work and feels her wages help to pay for the bills. She organises day care for the 4-year-old and has arranged her hours so that she is able to take the 6-year-old to and from school.

Both husband and wife are from Edinburgh and have a wide social network of friends and relatives about whom they say 'We can count on them.'

The present situation is a shock to both of them. Mr Royal refers to his stoma by waving his hand in the direction of his abdomen and saying, 'That thing'. Mrs Royal's reference is 'The operation'. The surgeon has told them that the colostomy will be permanent as the tumour was extensive but that he feels the surgery was successful in removing all of the contained tumour.

Summary of assessment

Client's questions/comments

---

1. How will 'this' affect my work?
2. I don't know what this means for travelling abroad in the future.
3. Is this thing really permanent?

Anticipated needs (research based)

Diagnosis—explained by Dr, needs to be followed up.
Treatment—needs to be explained.
Investigations—Dr to explain, nurse to detail.
Prognosis—good, informed by Dr.
Progress—individual previously healthy, non-smoker, moderate (3–4 beer/week) drinker, jogs (3 miles) daily. Expected to recover physical stamina quickly. Anticipated hospital stay—eight days.
Self-care—should progress to complete self-care
Routine—to be learned

Aids/barriers to learning

Aids—well educated, Mr Royal will be able to understand the discussions about his colostomy and learn self-care. As a science teacher he is accustomed to using manual skill to set up experiments and this will help him to manipulate the equipment used in stoma appliance management.

Barriers—the colostomy was not anticipated. Mr Royal is still shocked by the outcome of the surgery. His wife, a significant person in his life, has not yet accepted the colostomy.

His motivation to learn about self-care is low. He has expressed no curiosity as yet.

Date	Learning deficit	Learning need	Priority
27/03/85	non-acceptance of colostomy due to suddenness of surgery	to understand the reasons for the formation of the colostomy	1
27/03/85	does not know about the physical care of his colostomy due to inexperience	to learn the principles of care for his stoma	2

Planning

Learning need 1: To understand the reasons for the result of surgery

The plan is to increase Mr Royal's understanding of the reasons for the colostomy to help him towards acceptance of it. If he does not accept the results of surgery, he will not be motivated to learn about self-care.

Objectives: After teaching Mr Royal will:

Cognitive learning	Learning level	Teaching method & aids
1. locate the site of his tumour in the large intestine (after 3 post-operative days)	1. knowledge	1. book diagrams, one-to-one teaching
2. discuss the functioning of the large intestine in relation to his colostomy (after 3 post-operative days)	2. application	2. discussion, diagrams to follow functioning of bowel

Cognitive learning	Learning level	Teaching method & aids
3. identify when bowel movements in the colostomy are most likely to occur (after 3 post-operative days)	3. application	3. meet with dietician to discuss effects of certain foods; leaflets from the Colostomy Welfare Group

Affective learning	Learning level	Teaching method & aids
1. use the proper terminology to refer to his colostomy (by discharge)	1. receiving	1. be a role model and use proper terminology consistently
2. begin to discuss his feelings about the colostomy (by discharge)	2. responding	2. provide occasions for discussion — use privacy
3. discuss how the colostomy will affect his teaching activities, jogging, sex life (within 6 weeks)	3. valuing	3. introduce to ostomy association and others successfully coping with ostomies; provide opportunity and privacy for him to bring up subjects or to introduce subjects as possible areas of concern; include wife when possible; communicate this objective to Community Health Nurses

Learning need 2: To learn the principles of care for his stoma

The plan is to use a specific recording format designed by Ewing (1984) which summarises on one sheet all pertinent detail about Mr Royal and his progress in learning about the physical care of his stoma (see Fig. 8.1). The listed guidelines are, in fact, the objectives for meeting the learning need of self-care and the learning level will begin with Mr Royal being encouraged to develop appliance management or psychomotor skills (perception and set—see Table 3.1) and proceed to his using full self-care skills in which he is able to alter and innovate his use of stoma appliances (adaptation and origination). The nurse works through the helping methods with specific teaching strategies:

1. Acting: by doing the appliance management
2. Teaching: by demonstrating, explaining
3. Guiding: by encouraging return demonstration
4. Supporting: by watching, reinforcing
5. Promoting self-care: by praising, providing opportunity for independent care.

Implementation

Progress notes on Mr Royal illustrate how he is progressing with his learning needs.

Date	Learning need	Nursing action and results
27/03/85 1530 hrs	1	After the departure of his wife I approached Mr Royal, screened his bed and asked if I could check his colostomy site. I asked him how he felt about it and he replied that 'I feel a bit numb, as if it isn't quite true.' I asked him if he would look at the site so I could explain the words we use when describing it. He seemed to become interested and looked at the site with no apparent adverse reaction. (LKH)

Figure 8.1 Teaching plan for learning about stoma appliance management (Ewing, 1984)

GUIDELINES	CARE DETAILS									HELPING METHOD	PATIENT DETAILS
preparation of equipment	method – trolley, box									Acting – A	Name: Mr Jack Royal
preparation of patient	location, position, time									Teaching – T	Date of Birth: 21/10/48
removal of old appliance	method									Guiding – G	Diagnosis Cancer of the rectum
skin care	cleanser, drying agent									Supporting – S	Operation Laparotomy Colostomy 24 mths
skin protection	intact, damaged, broken									Home Care/ Self Care – SC	Type of stoma: ileostomy, colostomy ✓
selection of new appliance	effluent – fluid, firm; type, size									Developmental Environment Reminders	Site of stoma: ileum, ascending colon, transverse colon, descending colon, sigmoid colon ✓
preparation of appliance	method									privacy	Form of stoma: end, loop ✓, double barrel
application	angle, accessories, closure									Uninterrupted Care	Length of stoma: spout, flush ✓, retracted
disposal	method									Exposure of stoma only	Physical condition: eyesight ✓ noglasses, hearing ✓, manual deformity none, skin problems none
										Screening of patient Terminology	Home conditions: toilet facilities inside, ground floor; Means of disposal city rubbish collection
										Facial expression	
										No Gloves	

Date	Learning need	Nursing action and results
27/03/85 2030 hrs	1 2	Colostomy appliance required changing. I explained to Mr Royal the procedure and told him I would do the change but would tell him about each step. He responded, 'That is disgusting and smelly. You do what you want with it.' He sounded angry and refused to observe the appliance change procedure. (EC)

These notes indicate that Mr Royal is not meeting his learning needs as yet. The nurse's approach must be consistent and understanding. In the second progress note the nurse commented on both learning needs because they are inseparable in reality. At this point in time the nurse could discuss Mr Royal's needs with his wife and other members of the health care team and the objectives and teaching plan may change to accommodate the situation. Or, because this is still the first post-operative day and Mr Royal's reactions to his altered form of elimination are judged to be within normal limits, the nurse may continue with her teaching plan for another twenty-four hours.

EXAMPLE 2: HIGH SCHOOL FEMALE STUDENTS AND MENSTRUATION

Pertinent data

Target group: class of 20 secondary school female students
Age: 12–13 years
Topic: menstruation
School: single-sex institution located in West Royal, a middle-class neighbourhood.
Previous teaching: at age 9–10, in a class on health. Given a general introduction on the menarche.
Time allowed by school authorities: 3 hours

First session: February 21, 1985

As the local health visitor, I was asked to conduct a health teaching session on menstruation for a class of 20 female students, who, in a class with their registration teacher, related misinformation about their understanding of the menarche. I asked the school authorities for three one-hour sessions. The first session was planned as an assessment of the girls' knowledge and attitudes which would aid the organisation of the other sessions. Thus, the initial learning deficits and related learning needs were:

Learning deficit	Learning need	Priority
1. misinformed about menstruation	1. to understand the functioning of the body during menstruation	1
2. attitudes about menstruation have been negative ('the curse') due to misinformation and initial sources of information	2. to explore their own attitudes about menstruation and how these have been formed	2

Learning need 1: To understand the functioning of the body during menstruation

Objectives: By the end of the session each student will be able to:

Cognitive	Learning level	Teaching strategies
1. draw a diagram of the female reproductive system	knowledge	whole group; use board and coloured chalk; have handouts for them to label with organ names

Cognitive	Learning level	Teaching strategies
2. locate correctly the organs involved in menstruation	knowledge	whole group; use board and coloured chalk; have handouts for them to label with organ names
3. explain the normal menstrual cycle	comprehension	whole group; use board and coloured chalk
4. explain the hormonal changes occurring in menstruation	knowledge	use memory device to aid in remembering names of hormones
5. (for those who are menstruating) compare their own cycle with what has been presented	application	one-to-one at end of session

Learning need 2: To explore their own attitudes about menstruation and how these have been formed

Objectives: By the end of the session each student will be able to:

Affective	Learning level	Teaching strategies
1. state her initial reaction to hearing that she will be a menstruating female	responding	small group teaching—4 or 5 in each group. Set task of sharing with one another their experience. Report to whole group

Affective	Learning level	Teaching strategies
2. discuss the things she has heard other people say about menstruation	responding	present list of myths about menstruation (see Table 8.1). Add student contributions, have students debate each myth
3. name her primary informants	responding	No strategy
4. discuss others' ideas about menstruation in a non-judgemental fashion	responding	small group discussions with introduction about accepting others' experiences and feelings
5. react to situations which can occur when a female is menstruating	responding	have students list situations. Add to the list from Table 8.2 if necessary. Ask them to think of the worst that could happen

Table 8.1 Myths about menstruation

Women who are menstruating:
1. turn milk sour
2. stop bread rising
3. rust brass and iron
4. are unclean
5. must not exercise

6. must not wash their hair
7. ⎫
8. ⎬ student contributions
9. ⎪
10. ⎭

Table 8.2 Situations which can occur when menstruating

1. Buying sanitary towels or tampons from a male assistant at the chemist's.
2. Leaking through layers of clothing.
3. Staying in a friend's house and having the family dog find your used sanitary towel in the rubbish bin

4. Trying to explain to your new boyfriend that you are having menstrual cramping and do not want to swim today.
5. Opening your bag in a crowd and having a tampon fall out.
6. ⎫
7. ⎬ Student contributions
8. ⎭

Progress notes: February 21, 1985

This first session was a bit chaotic. I decided to begin by being practical and helping them to learn about the anatomy and physiology of the menstrual cycle. They are a very keen group and proved quite able to grasp and remember facts. Six of the girls are already menstruating and two of these are very knowledgeable. They were able to contribute very well to this first part of the session. The last half of the session which explored attitudes was very noisy with much laughter and teasing. However, since the affective objectives were met, the second half appeared to be successful. Further assessment of the group was done in this session and aids and barriers to learning were identified.

Aids. All the students have been achieving good results in school and their ability to participate in the fact-learning session was high. Some of the girls are menstruating and are willing to share their knowledge and/or experiences. They understand that this learning is important to them as females.

Barriers. The early adolescent stage the students are experiencing makes them act silly at times, thereby interrupting the session. The misinformation they have been exposed to persuades them to reject all other information initially, especially since the misinformation has originated from persons significant to them, e.g., mothers, favourite aunts or neighbours, older sisters. Owing to this, a certain amount of repetition will have to occur and this guides the second planning stage. The school authorities have decided they can give only two hours to this health teaching. Therefore, there is only one hour left.

Second session: February 28, 1985

In the first session, since I had not met the students, I decided to work on the learning need which the registration teacher had identified, namely a lack of correct knowledge about menstruation. The opportunity to explore attitudes helped to generate discussion and ease the atmosphere of slight embarrassment. In the second session I planned, first, to find out how much of the factual basis they remembered from the first session and, second, to elicit their learning needs as they defined them and to plan the last part of the session around their needs. Therefore, the learning deficits and related needs could not be set down prior to the session.

Objectives: By the end of the second session each student will be able to:

	Learning level	*Teaching strategies*
1. review the anatomy and physiology of the menstrual cycle as presented February 21, 1985	Cognitive— knowledge	oral quiz, using diagrams on overhead projector
2. list the areas related to menstruation about which she wants to know more	Cognitive— knowledge, comprehension	brainstorm for list of areas. Put student interest list on board to decide on topics (see Table 8.3)
3. participate in group discussions on the topics chosen	Affective— valuing	students to break into small groups to discuss specific topic

Table 8.3 Student interest list used to decide on topics

Students to indicate by voting which topics are most popular
1. Feminine hygiene_____
2. Toxic shock syndrome_____
3. Menstrual extraction_____
4. Menstruation and the pill_____
5. Dysmenorrhoea_____
6. Amenorrhoea_____
7. Gynaecological examination_____
8. Premenstrual tension_____
9.
10.

Progress notes:

The second session went well. The factual review demonstrated that most had learned the anatomy and physiology of the menstrual cycle. The problem area had to do with the hormonal changes. This was reinforced by going over the diagrams and memory device again. The brainstorming exercise pinpointed three areas of common concern: dysmenorrhoea, feminine hygiene including toxic shock syndrome, and premenstrual tension. Each area was discussed first by me. As an example, for dysmenorrhoea the following content was given:

Dysmenorrhoea or painful menstruation
—a common problem
—symptoms: pain, headaches, nausea, dizziness, backache, leg pain, faintness.
—Two kinds:
1. primary: in the absence of pelvic disease
2. secondary: in the presence of conditions like endometriosis.
—causes: many theories have been forwarded, eg, endocrine or hormonal imbalances; abnormal reproductive anatomy; psychogenic factors; present theory about prostaglandins.
—treatment:
1. pharmacological: use of analgesics, hormones
2. nonpharmacological: nutrition is important, decrease sodium intake, use natural diuretics to reduce fluid retention, exercise for muscle toning, mild heat, sleep and rest.

Students then met in small groups to compare notes on what they knew and how they coped (if menstruating) or have seen others cope (mothers, sisters, female relatives).

The discussion in this second session appeared to be much more serious with little laughing and giggling. Working with the students' self-identified needs increased their motivation and participation levels. Several students expressed interest in further meetings outside of school hours. This was arranged and all were invited to attend and bring friends and mothers if desired.

EXAMPLE 3: PRE-OPERATIVE PREPARATION

Ward 10 is a busy gynaecological ward with a rapid turnover of patients, the vast majority of whom are in hospital for three days or less. In response to this, a fairly routinised approach to pre-operative preparation has been developed. Clearly, this has disadvantages in individual cases, but the staff are convinced that the introduction of a systematic approach has been beneficial to both patients and staff. There has been no formal evaluation, since it has proved beyond their resources (both time and perhaps expertise) to design adequate outcome measures.

A previously successful venture in patient education had been the development of written sheets giving information to patients about their self-care on discharge from hospital. These were prepared jointly by the nursing and medical staff. Devising a systematic approach to pre-operative care seemed the next logical step in the development of nursing practice. The medical staff had no objections, and indeed welcomed the proposals.

Assessment

It was decided that since large numbers of women pass through the ward each year, undergoing a limited range of surgical operations, it would be relatively simple to produce a list of anticipated information needs in relation to each type of operation. In the event, we have been able to categorise and group certain surgical operations, because patients have very similar experiences and information needs. This case study describes the work done in relation to preparing patients to undergo laparoscopy for sterilisation purposes. Figure 8.2 shows the checklist of anticipated needs which was agreed by nursing and medical staff. It was decided that the nurse who prepared the patient for theatre should spend five to ten minutes discussing these items with every patient. Since then we have split this into two short sessions, as is shown on the teaching plan which follows.

We were also aware of the dangers of taking a standard approach to the individual, and so it was decided that there would be some attempt at assessing individual needs on admission. This is done by allowing a few minutes for discussion of the forthcoming surgery, and by recording the woman's questions and comments. These are taken as indicators of possible aids or barriers to learning, and an attempt is made to note the specific issues of concern to the patient. The as-

---

Ward 10   Pre-operative information (sterilisation)

Diagnosis — Check known and understood

Treatment
1. Doctor will carry out a general physical examination the evening before surgery
2. The patient's husband will be required to sign consent for the sterilisation
3. Nothing must be taken by mouth after 10.00 pm the evening before surgery
4. Bathing is required in the morning before going to theatre
5. A 'bikini line' shave will be carried out
6. A pre-medication is given before theatre
7. The nurse who gives the pre-medication will (as necessary) remove dentures, contact lenses and hairgrips and tape rings to fingers
8. There will be two small abdominal incisions with clips

Progress / self-care
9. The patient will 'come to' in the anaesthetic room
10. A cup of tea and toast will be given once the patient is awake
11. The clips will most likely be removed immediately before discharge
12. There may be shoulder pain post-operatively because of gas used to distend the abdominal cavity to allow the surgeon to view the reproductive organs with a telescope-like instrument
13. The patient should stay off work for two days following discharge

Ward layout / routine
14. Whereabouts of television room (smoking permitted immediately after meals)
15. Valuables have to be locked away

Figure 8.2 Checklist of pre-operative teaching needs

sessment data are summarised. Figure 8.3 shows the summary sheet for a 32-year-old school teacher (Mrs Jones) admitted for laparoscopy.

Learning needs

Generally, these are assumed to be the 15 information items (Fig. 8.2) but special note is made of individual differences, such as:

1. the expressed fear of pain and
2. expressed desire to smoke, as in Mrs Jones' case.

Name: Mrs Jean Jones **Age:** 32 years **Diagnosis:** Laparoscopy for sterilisation purposes **Personal data:** stable marriage, 2 children	

Patient's questions/comments
How long will I be off work? Can I smoke in here? I'm an awful coward about pain

Anticipated needs (research based)	
Diagnosis Treatment Investigations Prognosis Progress Self-care Routine	(See pre-prepared checklist)

Aids/barriers to Learning	
Age Cognitive state Educational level Emotional level – Grasp of technical – language Hearing Comfort Previous experience Sex Motivation to learn Attitude Learning ability	Some apprehension, but otherwise no difficulties anticipated 15 items of information, but reasonably straightforward

Figure 8.3   Summary of assessment data

Planning

Because there are large numbers of patients requiring pre-operative preparation for very similar operations each week, in-dividual objectives are not always written. In all instances, there is the expectation that patients:

1. must be able to recall items 3 and 13
2. should be able to recall other information about treatment and pre-operative care.

In Mrs Jones' case there would be further objectives related to fear of pain and smoking.

Teaching plan

This would be detailed in the nursing notes as follows:

Timing	Staff member	Objectives	Method	Outcome
Thurs. pm, following anaesthetist's visit	S/N Harris	1,2	discussion + *categorise and order* information items	
Wed. am, prior to discharge	S/N Smith	1, item 13		

The teaching task is considered to be straightforward, and the plan does not allow for involvement of more than two members of staff in any formal sense, though it is recognised that individual patients may ask questions of any staff member at any time, and they are encouraged to do so. It is also made clear that there is time set aside for patients to ask questions and that both an anaesthetist and a nurse would be coming to discuss the operation with the patient prior to surgery.

Implementation

It is generally assumed that most people have at least some fears and worries about surgery, and the pre-operative teaching session is geared to allaying anxiety as well as to imparting information. Attempts are made to ensure that the session, which usually lasts only five or ten minutes, will be uninterrupted and is as private as possible.

There is no formula for success. Perhaps the most important single concern for the nurse is to attempt to listen carefully to what the woman has to say, and to avoid assuming knowledge of her thoughts and feelings. A useful approach might be to begin the discussion as follows:

> I am Staff Nurse Harris and I am here to talk with you about going to theatre tomorrow. There are one or two things I

want you to remember, but first tell me how you are feeling about it.' This open-ended approach may help her to express fears and worries. If it doesn't — for instance, if she says 'I am OK' — then it is a matter of judgement as to whether it is helpful to probe further at this stage. Sometimes it helps to accept such a reply at face value and to proceed to give the information items as planned. The very act of being willing to provide information, as well as the information itself, may allay anxiety. In some instances it may be helpful to make reference to the individual's expressed concerns. In Mrs Jones' case, for instance, the fear of pain might be explored.

To assist recall, it may help to order and categorise information items. The essential items 3 and 13 would usually be given first. A useful categorisation for other items might be 'things which happen before you go to theatre' and 'things which happen after you have had the operation'.

Evaluation

There is no formal attempt at ascertaining outcomes, in terms either of patients' increased satisfaction with information or of lessened anxiety, because of the measurement difficulties posed. In any case, previous research (Hayward, 1975; Boore, 1978) appears to have established that there are benefits. The

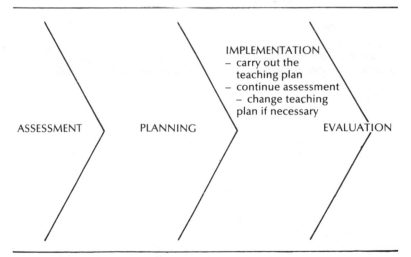

Figure 8.4 The implementation process

nursing notes include a column in which staff record subjective impressions of the outcome of teaching, and note any unusual aspects of the communication process.

The examples presented in this chapter were developed to illustrate how, in the implementation phase, assessment, planning and evaluation are on-going processes which can redirect the focus of the health teacher and learner. Figure 8.4 shows where the implementation process fits in teaching and learning.

REFERENCES

Boore J R P 1978 Prescription for recovery. Royal College of Nursing, London
Ewing G 1984 A study of the postoperative nursing care of stoma patients during appliance changes. Unpublished doctoral dissertation, University of Edinburgh
Fogel C A, Woods N F 1981 Health care of women: a nursing perspective. C V Mosby Company, London
Hayward J 1975 Information: a prescription against pain. Royal College of Nursing, London
McPherson A, Anderson A 1983 Women's problems in general practice. Oxford University Press, Oxford
Smith E D 1981 Women's health care: a guide for patient education. Appleton-Century-Crofts, New York

FURTHER READING

Anderson D C 1979 Health education in practice. Croom Helm, London
Bennett A E (ed) 1976 Communication between doctors and patients. Nuffield Provincial Hospitals Trust, Oxford University Press, London

9

Evaluation of
health teaching

OBJECTIVES

Study of this chapter will enable you to:

1. Discuss the importance of planned evaluation.
2. Describe what is meant by evaluation.
3. Distinguish types of evaluation.
4. Discuss the limitations of evaluation designs.
5. Discuss the appropriate use of various techniques of evaluation.
6. Consider the value of feedback.

Evaluation is an inevitable part of the teaching—learning process. Whether or not the teacher plans for it to happen both learner and teacher will evaluate. The learner may say 'that was helpful' or 'that was nonsense' or 'I see what she means, but . . .'. These are all evaluative statements. The teacher may say 'I did that well', or 'I made that very complicated' or 'I explained that quite well, except for.. . .'. Again, these are evaluative statements.

Such subjective evaluation can be useful, but it has obvious limitations. Both teacher and learner need more detailed and constructive feedback. The teacher should not be content with an intuitive sense that all went well, but should attempt to identify exactly what has been achieved. Likewise, the learner should aim to assess his grasp of new knowledge, or acceptance of the ideas proposed.

In a good teaching and learning environment, intuitive assessment will be replaced by a more planned approach. Both teacher and learner may have to develop the skills of planned evaluation. In some situations they may even do this jointly. For example, in cases of psychiatric illness or spinal cord injury, where rehabilitation is a complex and long-term process, both nurse and patient have much to learn together, and will develop skills in setting goals and assessing outcomes as part of that process of learning. More usually, however, the nurse, as teacher, will assist the patient or client, as learner, to acquire the relevant skills.

THE BENEFITS OF PLANNED EVALUATION

Planned evaluation is an important part of the health teaching process for a number of reasons. Firstly, it gives tangible evidence of what has been accomplished. This motivates the learner and helps the nurse gain job satisfaction and confidence in her teacher role. Secondly, evaluation provides the means to weigh achievement against stated goals. This allows the possibility of planned future improvements. Every teaching programme has to be adjusted to the individual learner, the talents of the teacher and the environment in which teaching takes place. Often such adjustment is immediate, in response to learner needs within a given teaching opportunity. Such spontaneous and often intuitive adjustment may, however, be backed by a planned and documented approach to evaluation. Sometimes it is only by reflecting upon the teaching process in retrospect that useful feedback can be provided. Planned evaluation exercises should incorporate the learner's views along with the teacher's, and make intuitive reactions subject to a degree of objectivity, perhaps even measurement.

A third reason for evaluating is to provide evidence that health teaching is worthwhile, in terms of what it costs. Sometimes this is a relatively easy exercise. For instance, recent research (Hayward, 1975; Boore, 1978) has demonstrated that giving information to patients as a preparation for surgery has proved to be beneficial in reducing the amount of analgesia required and the incidence of post-operative infection. It is possible to calculate such benefits and thus demonstrate the *cost benefit* of health education. Rocella (1976) has described a range of examples of cost beneficial health education. It should be noted, however, that health education, along with many other aspects of health care, cannot always be justified on economic grounds alone. Health education in the prevention of heart disease provides a good example of this problem since it can be argued that it might be cheaper to let people die of coronary artery disease than to sustain the costs of care in old age.

That particular equation is very complicated. How are costs of lost production to be estimated? Or the costs of a teenager losing a father? Besides, health educators might argue (though with little or no proof at present) that health education can contribute to a fitter and more independent old age, thus reducing costs of caring for the elderly.

Despite the difficulties, there are increasing demands, in times of financial stringency, to demonstrate the benefits of health education in financial terms, and this aspect of evaluation should be a primary concern of anyone planning for health teaching. Indeed, planners may require the individual health educator to demonstrate not only that health education makes financial sense in relation to other aspects of health care, but that the particular programme of health education recommended is *cost effective*. A cost-effective programme is one which achieves the health care objectives most efficiently, in other words, at similar or less cost than other programmes achieving comparable results.

Other reasons for carrying out evaluation reflect social and emotional as well as practical considerations. For instance, if health teaching is to mean the difference between feeling well and being very ill, as in severe diabetes mellitus, then evaluation of the extent of learning, in this case about the use of insulin, diet and energy expenditure, will be essential. At the end of the day, the issue of how health teaching benefits the recipient may be as important as the consideration of costs. Being pain-free in the post-operative stage sooner than the average patient, is likely to be more important to the individual concerned than is any reduction in the cost of analgesia. Evaluation of the usefulness of health education should thus be geared to the recipient's as well as the planner's view of utility.

The nurse who evaluates her health teaching demonstrates her willingness to be held accountable for it. She is able to show, through judgement which may incorporate measurement, whether her efforts were effective. If learning has not occurred, evaluation helps to pinpoint reasons and provides the basis of re-assessment from which further planning, teaching and evaluation may proceed.

DEFINING EVALUATION

Evaluation, then, is a planned process and should be continuous; it is made in regard to stated criteria, which may be developed and applied by both teacher and learner, and may involve measurement.

The steps in evaluation are:

1. Consider the objectives of the health teaching.
2. Identify the object of interest for the evaluation: knowledge, attitudes or behaviour.
3. Design the evaluation programme.
4. Select or devise measurements.
5. Collect and analyse data.
6. Present the results, and provide feedback.

Educationalists (Bloom et al, 1971; Guilbert, 1977) distinguish *formative* and *summative* evaluation. The term 'formative' is applied to evaluation used as a continuous process of feedback throughout the teaching and learning situation. This type of evaluation helps to determine the pace and extent of learning and allows the health teacher to vary teaching activity to meet the learner's needs. Formative evaluation is a mechanism which enhances the teaching–learning situation. In this way it is different from the 'summative' evaluation which is done at the end of a teaching–learning programme specifically to identify how much has been learned. Most people have experienced summative evaluation in the form of final school exams which determine whether or not one progresses to another educational level, and it may be for this reason that evaluation is often assumed to be concerned only with end results. However, both types of evaluation are necessary in health teaching, and in this text the distinction between types of evaluation is further refined by use of three terms which are now used fairly commonly in health care evaluation. These are: structure, process and outcome.

AREAS OF EVALUATION—STRUCTURE, PROCESS, OUTCOME

Structure, process and outcome are three areas of evaluation which help to analyse the who, what and how of the health education process (see Fig. 9.1). Comprehensive evaluation will encompass all three areas.

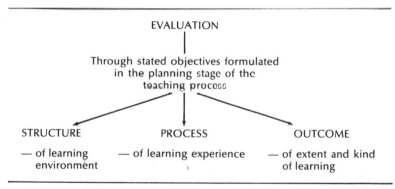

Figure 9.1 Comprehensive evaluation includes consideration of structure, process and outcome measures.

Structure

Evaluation of structure is concerned with aspects of the learning environment including the availability and use of such factors as premises, expertise, equipment and manpower. Structural evaluation is characterised by consideration of the availability and accessibility of teaching and looks at what is organised for teaching. In a hospital setting the concern might be with provision of privacy or timing of post discharge instructions. In the community, structural evaluation might aim at determining whether the location of the clinic where classes were held was influential in encouraging people to attend or whether the supply of audio-visual equipment gave ease of access to all. Additionally, structural evaluation relates to such activities as recording the details of topics covered, the numbers attending and with monitoring the expressed satisfaction of learners.

This type of evaluation is necessary to good planning, but it has limitations. It is not enough to know that there was a good turn out at a health education film or that most people seemed satisfied. Equally, information about the proportion of patients who received pre-operative instruction and which members of staff were involved, is of little use in the absence of any evidence of the success of such instruction.

Evaluation of structure—some guiding questions

1. What topics were dealt with?
2. Which staff were involved?
3. Were the facilities and resources adequate?
4. Was there enough time?
5. Was the environment conducive to learning?
6. Did people seem satisfied?

Process

Evaluation of process deals with how resources are used, which type of technique was employed and how appropriate were these resources and techniques in relation to the par-ticular learner and the learning task in hand. Such evaluation is a joint venture between the health teacher and the learner.

In a way, what is being analysed is the art of teaching. How did it happen? How was it organised? This is the act of relating the subject matter and the objectives to a series of tasks and activities. The term process refers to what happens between teacher and learner. Setting out to help a person to learn how to inject himself involves visualising the end result and plan-ning teaching in stages which will achieve that result. The likely approach is to use demonstration or a film to show the technique of injection, then break the skill into a set of subroutines. At each point, various methods and techniques are available to reinforce learning. Choice of these, along with everything else which occurs, may help or hinder the learning experience. Thus the process of learning and teaching should be recorded fully to allow examination of positive and negative influences on learning. An example of process recording technique is given in Figure 9.6.

The essence of good process evaluation is to provide for constructive feedback, throughout the learning and at the end. Without the facility for feedback throughout, learning may proceed slowly and inefficiently. The learner will experience a certain amount of intrinsic feedback in the act of learning. However, his own assessment is seldom enough and constructive comment from the health teacher is essential to motivation. In some instances it may be necessary to help the learner identify and acknowledge his attainments. The quality of the assessment and the way it is given are important considerations: feedback should be informative, reinforcing and motivating.

Evaluation of process—some guiding questions

The learner
Were the learner's perceptions of his need for health teaching elicited?
Was the learner involved in the selection of learning method?
How did the learner participate?
Were there fluctuations in the level of participation?
What kind of responses did the learner make?

The health teacher
Was the teacher credible to the learners?
Which teaching style was used, and was it appropriate?
Did the teacher relate positively to the learners?
Was the interaction active and was discussion allowed?
Was the teacher organised, consistent, accepting and respectful of the learner; a listener; provider of feedback; knowledgeable?

The method
Were the methods used for health teaching learner-centred or teacher-centred?

Did these methods build on experience and ability?
Were the learners motivated and stimulated by the methods?

The content
Was the content logically organised?
Was the amount right?
Did the content relate to the learner's previous knowledge and experience?

The objectives
Were the objectives specific, realistic and meaningful in relation to the health education needs of the individual?

Outcome

Evaluation of outcome is concerned with end results. For this some kind of measure is usually required. The desired outcomes of health teaching may be defined as changes in knowledge, attitudes and behaviour. It is a necessary first step in evaluation to clarify the purpose of the health education programme, in order to identify suitable outcome measures. If the programme seeks to influence behaviour, then measures of changed knowledge or attitude will not suffice, since it can be demonstrated that the link between knowledge, attitudes and behaviour is uncertain. Equally, it is unrealistic, and unfair, to apply measures of behavioural outcome to a programme designed only to change knowledge or awareness.

Measurements of attitude change are difficult both to construct and to apply. For this reason, and perhaps because the link between attitudes and behaviour has been in some doubt, measures of health teaching outcome are commonly sought in relation to knowledge factors or to behaviour.

Instruments to measure knowledge are fairly easily constructed but may be difficult to apply. Adults, whether in hospital, attending a family planning clinic, a series of pre-natal classes or a single lecture on the causes of alcoholism, may find knowledge questionnaires threatening or even insulting.

The measurement of behaviour presents a considerable challenge: behavioural outcomes vary in the extent to which they are observable and amenable to reliable recording. Table 9.1 outlines some of the options. Some behavioural outcomes may be observed, recorded and measured readily. The use of

Table 9.1 Some health indicators

Vital	Health actions
Birth rate	· Use of services
Mortality	Preventive actions
Population growth	Consumption patterns
Social	Disease
Illegitimacy	Morbidity
Unemployment	Disability
Absenteeism	Restriction to activity

a specific service such as chiropody is an example. Vital indicators, such as morbidity, mortality and fertility, are also readily available, though negative, health indices. Others, such as preventive actions, consumption patterns or compliance with prescribed drug regimens, are less easily observed. In such cases, recording may depend on self-reports and clearly these are subject to bias. Some indicators such as illegitimacy, unemployment and absenteeism are easily recorded but less easily interpreted in health terms. There have been attempts at producing reliable health indices which will reflect social, emotional and physical functioning (Culyer, 1983) but there is a long way to go before indices are developed which will satisfy the needs of health care planners and reflect experiences and views of health seen as relevant by members of the public.

Setting evaluation criteria

If the purpose of evaluation is to weigh achievement against aims then it will be necessary to establish criteria for judging success. In individualised patient education, the instructional objectives, if properly written, will specify these, and this can be done in negotiation with the patient. In community-based programmes, however, it may be more difficult to establish what change in knowledge or behaviour constitutes success.

Somehow, a standard has to be set. Green (1974) looked at a number of studies and identified different standards of acceptability for patient education outcomes. One of these was the *absolute standard* wherein the standard is set by policy makers who have opted for an unrealistic 100% solution. Equally unsatisfactory is the *arbitrary standard*, based upon whim or hunch. Sometimes it is possible to establish an *historical standard*, by looking at trends relating to the individual's personal history, the population at risk or the health problem. The use of *normative standards* involves comparison with the outcomes of programmes carried out for similar reasons, with like populations in similar environments. This provides a sounder basis for standard setting as does the use of *theoretical standards* or those based on predictions from theory or on previous research. Sometimes a *negotiated standard* can be set in which the desired change in behaviour is jointly determined, as can happen in care managed on the basis of a contract between professionals and patients.

Evaluation of outcome—some guiding questions

The learner
What were the changes in knowledge and/or behaviour?
Was there any evidence of an increased ability to analyse, to participate, to adapt health actions?
Did the learner consider he benefited?

The health teacher
Did the teacher's health knowledge or behaviour change?
Were insights into health-related behaviour gained?

The method
Did it achieve the desired results?
Was it more economical than other comparable methods?

The objectives
Were they achievable?
Were they measurable? By which standards?
Were they met?
Whose objectives were met?

EVALUATION DESIGNS FOR OUTCOME ASSESSMENT

One of the challenges of recording the outcomes of health teaching is to find adequate and positive indices of health. In addition, even where acceptable and reliable outcome measures exist, it may be difficult to establish that any change in health-related knowledge or behaviour can be attributed to the particular health teaching intervention. Careful choice of an experimental or quasi-experimental research design will help.

Consider four common evaluation designs, shown in Figure 9.2. In *design 1* the only observations or measurements occurred after the health teaching. Therefore, the evaluation cannot determine whether or not there has been any change in the learner's knowledge level or health behaviour.

	Key:	X = teaching		
		O = observation		
1. Post-test only		X O_1		
2. Pre-and post-test		O_1 X O_2		
3. Using a control group	Experimental group	O_1	X	O_2
	Control group	O_1		O_2
4. Random allocation of persons into groups	Experimental group	R	X	O_1
	Control group	R		O_2

Figure 9.2 Four evaluation designs

Design 2, because it was a pre-test, is more useful, but there are limitations. It does not allow for changes which might have occurred over time in any case: subjects may have matured; they may have been influenced by another educational experience such as a television programme. It is also possible that the pre-test influenced the post-test, though this is less of a concern in health teaching than it would be in pure research, since pre-testing is often part of the teaching strategy and may be used to motivate learners.

Design 3 utilises the concept of *control* as a way around the problems found in the pre-and post-test design. Use of control groups can help isolate the effects of the health teaching intervention. This design requires that the experimental group are taught and tested. The control group are tested along with them but not taught. This offers some improvement, but again there are limitations because the pre-test does not establish everything about the groups. It has to be assumed that they are comparable. In pure research this problem can be minimised by careful choice of control and statistical application with sufficiently large samples. In health education, however, this presents problems in practice because it may mean using a questionnaire type of evaluation with possible resulting superficiality of data. It may also mean that the health teaching to be applied is equally superficial, in order to achieve adequately-sized samples. The research phenomenon that it is possible to achieve either a large representative sample with superficial data or a data-rich study carried out in a sample which is either small, or has no adequate control group, presents a particular challenge to the health educator (Green, 1977).

Design 4 offers one solution to the problem of finding a research design which will demonstrate conclusively the effects of any teaching intervention. The answer lies in using randomly allocated learners. This fourth design is similar to the third one, but the random allocation of subjects into groups means that initial differences in the two groups are equalised by randomisation. In terms of the research problem this is a neat solution. For the health educator, however, some difficulties remain. It may not be easy to achieve random allocation of people into groups. This is particularly the case in community education where groups are often self-selecting. This design can, however, be applied where groups are convened by health educators (for example, pre-natal classes) who thus have control over the flow of members. It may also be applicable in patient education, provided any ethical issues about the withholding of information can be resolved.

TECHNIQUES OF EVALUATION

Techniques of evaluation help to gather information which, when interpreted, assess if and how learning has occurred. As has been stressed, the techniques must be designed to measure the kind or kinds of learning specified in the objectives for the educational programme. Two qualities of measurement are additional essential considerations, *validity* and *reliability*.

When a method or technique of measurement is valid, it has measured what it was intended to assess. For instance, assessing the effects of senior citizens' exercise programmes on flexibility of movement by giving a written questionnaire would be an invalid method. Observing exercises in progress or actually measuring how much the senior citizens can flex and extend limbs would be a valid approach.

The second term, reliability, refers to the consistency of a measurement tool. If a health visitor concerned with the incidence of ischaemic heart disease in the community, tested the knowledge level of her clients about the health risks of smoking, the results should be the same on one day as on the next. That is, the tool should generate consistent responses provided there has been no intervening teaching or experience to change their knowledge.

A wide range of evaluation techniques is available. Figure 9.3 indicates how they might be applied in the evaluation of structure, process and outcome.

Oral questioning

This is a readily available, and thus important, tool for the health teacher, for in most nursing situations the evaluation of learning may need to be on-going and immediate. Questioning is a central critical element in health teaching because it promotes thinking about the subject under discussion. In evaluation, questioning permits the health teacher to check comprehension, to test knowledge, and to diagnose weaknesses in the learner's knowledge base. How the questions are posed is important. Chapter 4 reviews therapeutic communication and provides guidelines about formulating questions. It is important to remember that the value of oral questioning as an evaluation technique will be enhanced in many instances if answers are recorded.

Questionnaire surveys

These have a useful but limited application in relation to

Evaluation area	Oral Questioning	Questionnaire Survey	Checklist	Rating scale	Written tests	Diaries	Process recording	Nursing audit
I STRUCTURE								
1. Facilities, resources, time allocation	X	X	X	X				X
2. Learning aids	X	X	X	X				X
II. PROCESS								
1. Participation and response of learner	X		X	X		X	X	
2. Health teacher characteristics			X	X		X		
3. Effectiveness of methods utilised	X		X	X				
4. Content organisation			X	X				X
III. OUTCOME								
1. Learning accomplished	X			X	X	X		
2. Teacher insight increased			X	X		X		
3. Goal and objective achievement				X	X	X		X
4. Programme value				X			X	X

Evaluation technique (column group heading)

Figure 9.3 Evaluation techniques used to assess the structure, process and outcome of the teaching-learning situation.

evaluation of structural factors and learner satisfaction. Good survey forms often look deceptively simple, but achieving validity and reliability can be difficult. Each question should be carefully considered, and pilot-tested. Useful further reading on this and every other technique in this section is noted at the end of this chapter.

Checklists

These are quite commonly used in patient education, usually as a reminder of content to be included. They also have a role to play in evaluation. Figure 9.4 shows two checklists. The first might be used in process evaluation, to check the content of pre-operative teaching. The second could be applied as an outcome measure to indicate whether someone with a newly formed colostomy has grasped the sequence involved in an appliance change. This checklist provides a reminder of the

Pre-operative information checklist
Information items

Signing of operation consent
Visit from the anaesthetist
Arrangements for fasting
Timing of surgery
Timing of pre-medication
Activity following pre-medication
Emptying of bladder
Removal of items: Jewellery
hair clips
dentures

Anaesthetic room procedure
Recovery
Visiting
Details of anticipated surgery
Post-operative
  expectations: – IV
              – drains
              – position
              – food and fluids
              – activity

Stoma care appliance change checklist

Action sequence

	Patient followed sequence	
	Yes	No
1. Chose location for change	✓	
2. Gathered equipment	✓	
3. Removed old appliance	✓	
4. Inspected skin area		✓
5. Provided skin care		✓
6. Measured stoma	✓	
7. Fitted new appliance	✓	
8. Tidied up	✓	

Figure 9.4 Checklists for (a) pre-operative preparation and (b) stoma appliance change.

sequence and evidence that the learner is following it except for inspecting the skin area and providing skin care. This would be a point for discussion.

Rating scales

These have their origins in psychological research. Traditionally they were used to assess attitudes. A typical rating scale consisted of a list of statements of opinion, against which people indicated their level of agreement in such terms as 'strongly agree', 'agree', 'disagree', 'strongly disagree'. Rating scales may be widely applied in the evaluation of health teaching: assessing the level of learner satisfaction, the effectiveness of methods used, and the extent of behavioural change are just three possible applications. Figure 9.5 shows how a rating scale item might be constructed to assess skill learning related to stoma care.

Objective:

The client inspects and describes the condition of the area of skin around the stoma with each change:

1	2	3
did not inspect skin condition	looked at area briefly did not describe skin condition	carefully examined skin area around stoma and described condition

---

Figure 9.5 Rating scale item

Written tests

These have wide application in some forms of health teaching, for instance, they may be applied within a school health education programme. In many situations, however, particularly in patient education, a written test will provide an unnecessary threat and so they should be used with care.

Some questions can help guide the construction of written tests:

1. Is the material worth a test?
2. Is this the best way of evaluating what has been learned?
3. Is the test at the reading and comprehension level of the learner?
4. Are the directions clear?
5. Has unnecessary jargon been avoided?

Below are examples of items which might be used to make up a written test:

True or False: The statements below are either true or false. Note in the space provided before each statement whether you believe it is true (T) or false (F).

1. ＿＿Ischaemic heart disease is one of the most common causes of death in Britain.
2. ＿＿Of developed countries, Japan has the lowest rate of ischaemic heart disease.

Fill in the blank: In each statement below a word is missing. Fill in the word you believe correctly completes the statement.

1. In a baby bath demonstration it must be remembered to proceed from clean areas to ＿＿.

2. While cleaning the baby's umbilical cord stump each day you should be particularly aware of _____.

Matching: Below are two columns of words. From the right column select words which are related to those in the left column. Enter the letter of the right column word beside the number of the left hand column word.

1. _____diabetic diet   a. type of carbohydrate
2. _____keto acidosis   b. urinary symptoms
3. _____symptom of undiagnosed   c. before lunch
         diabetes
4. _____common hypoglycaemia   d. acetone on breath
         attacks

Multiple choice: Below are statements or questions followed by a selection of possible answers. Select the answer you feel is correct by circling the letter preceding the answer.

1. When a diabetic person has missed a meal, a possible repercussion might be:
   a. Ketoacidosis
   b. Hyperglycaemia
   c. Hypoglycaemia
   d. Hypertension

Diaries

These also provide useful material for evaluation. They can be used by both health teacher and learner to record personal observations about their own reactions and feelings to a teaching—learning situation. The entries are then compared and analysed for changes in attitude and feelings and even behaviour. Learner diaries can be used to assess the reaction to the structure and process of the learning situation. Teacher diaries may provide insight for the individual nurse as to her own feelings and reactions.

Process recordings

These can help to analyse the effectiveness of the teaching—learning process. Figure 9.6 illustrates how a process recording can assist examination of the content and feeling of the interaction between the learner and health teacher. Mr

What the patient said and did (verbal and nonverbal communication)	What the nurse said and did	Analysis
	I noticed from the chart that Mr Hughes, a patient with a recent colostomy, had not begun to learn how to care for his stoma. I decided to assess his readiness for learning. I went to his bed on the ward, introduced myself, and said, 'Mr Hughes, I see you have had a colostomy and that the nurses have been changing the appliance for you.'	This was the first time I had met Mr Hughes. Perhaps it might have been better to have one of the nurses who has been caring for him make the approach. I noted his immediate reticence but decided to proceed. I may have made him guilty by the way I opened the conversation.
Looked uncomfortable. Replied 'yes.' Not volunteering anything else.		
	'Do you have any questions about the colostomy?'	
'No.' Sounded angry.		
		'Tell me what has been happening with your colostomy?' *or* 'How do you feel you are getting on?' Might have been better as a first question.

Figure 9.6 Illustration of a process recording

Hughes does not appear to be ready to proceed with learning about colostomy care. The nurse considers whether or not her approach was a contributing factor in Mr Hughes' response.

Nursing audits

These may provide the context of health teaching evaluation. The function of a nursing audit is to determine the level of care given and to provide evidence of the success or failure of nursing care. Nursing audits may be accomplished by a single nurse, but more usually a peer group or the care team will peruse nursing care plans to determine the adequacy of care.

The health teaching strengths of the nursing team may be built up through the process of nursing audit. The essence of the audit is to provide time to reflect upon the assumed purposes, the process and the outcome of health teaching in a given environment, be it ward, clinic, health centre, school, industrial premises or whatever. The audit operates by providing opportunities for constructive feedback. Patients, clients, and the entire care team may have a part to play in this learning process from time to time. However, on a day-to-day basis, the audit will be managed by the nursing staff and much of the activity will centre upon detailed examination of the nursing care plan. In relation to health teaching, teaching plans can be perused to identify a number of factors:

1. How did the plan proceed?
2. Did the learner achieve the objectives? To what extent?
3. How did the nurses record teaching sessions? Is the recording easily understood?

Clearly, the adequacy of documentation will be vital to the process of audit. One concern is to produce a see-at-a-glance record which will enable progress to be identified quickly. Figure 9.7 shows one such format which a nurse researcher has developed from research on stoma appliance management (Ewing, 1984). The teaching plan for the patient is based upon a self-care perspective. Thus the helping methods are progressive, with the nurse acting (A) for the learner in the first instance, teaching (T) when he is ready, guiding him (G) in his learning, supporting him (S) when he does the procedure and assessing when he is completely self-caring (SC). The left hand column (guidelines) presents a reminder of the steps in care which are to be taught, while the next column records current details of the prescribed care. The dated columns indicate clearly that on Day One the nurse did all his stoma care for the patient, on Days Two and Three she began teaching him. By the sixth day he is managing with support, but he has not yet achieved self-care. If this situation still pertained on the day of discharge a nursing audit might reveal

GUIDELINES	CARE DETAILS	9/9/84	10/9/84	11/9/84	13/9/84	14/9/84	15/9/84		HELPING METHOD	PATIENT DETAILS
preparation of equipment	method – trolley box to ward bathroom	A	A	AT	G	G	SC		Acting – A Teaching – T	Name: Ms Leslie Hardy Date of Birth: 09/03/47
preparation of patient	location ward bathroom position sitting time usually after breakfast	A	AT	AT	G	G	SC		Guiding – G Supporting – S	Diagnosis Cancer of cervix Operation Laparotomy Colostomy
removal of old appliance	method gentle peel	A	AT	AT	G	G	SC		Home Care/Self Care – SC	Type of stoma: ileostomy colostomy ✓
skin care	cleanser soap + H2O drying agent none	A	AT	AT	AT	G	G			Site of stoma: ileum ascending colon transverse colon descending colon sigmoid colon ✓
skin protection	intact ✓ from 9/9/84 damaged use cream paste broken stoma adhesive	A	AT	AT	AT	G	G		Developmental Environment Reminders	
selection of new appliance	effluent – fluid firm type coloplast and size drainable 40	A	A	AT	G	G	SC		privacy ✓	Form of stoma: end loop ✓ double barrel
preparation of appliance	method measure with guide, cut and peel	A	A	AT	AT	G	SC		Uninterrupted Care ✓	Length of stoma: spout flush ✓ retracted
application	angle vertical accessories belt closure surgical clips	A	A	AT	AT	G	SC		Exposure of stoma only ✓	
									Screening of patient ✓ Terminology understands terms	Physical condition: eyesight slight myopia uses glasses hearing good manual deformity none skin problems none
disposal	method ward toilet	A	A	AT	G	G	SC		Facial expression accepting No Gloves	Home conditions: toilet facilities bathroom Means of disposal

Figure 9.7 Teaching plan for learning about stoma appliance management (Ewing, 1984) showing use in evaluation.

that the teaching process had not progressed sufficiently. This, then, would be a case for discussion.

WHO NEEDS FEEDBACK?

Much of this chapter has centered on feedback: what it is, why we need it, how to provide it, what to do with it. We have dealt with three aspects:

Feedback for the learner: which will motivate and guide learning.

Feedback for the teacher: which will indicate strengths and weaknesses, allowing for improvements in teaching and for job satisfaction.

Feedback for managers and health care planners: which will help identify effective use of health teaching and thus inform the planning process.

In the end, if the learner has achieved the objectives set in the planning stage and is able to demonstrate the ability to use health knowledge to analyse his health problems and potential, to adopt behaviours which promote optimum living, and to hold positive attitudes about such behaviour, then the teaching process may be deemed effective.

However, if the objectives have not been achieved, the evaluation may help to determine the reasons and the process of teaching begins again with an assessment which may change the plans and actions of the participants so that health teaching becomes an effective tool in the promotion of healthy living.

REFERENCES

Boore J 1978 Prescription for recovery. Royal College of Nursing, London
Bloom B S, Hastings J T, Madaus G F 1971 Handbook on formative and summative evaluation of student learning. McGraw-Hill Book Company, Toronto.
Culyer A J (ed) 1983 Health indicators: an international study for the European Science Foundation. Martin Robertson and Company Ltd, Oxford
Ewing G 1984 A study of the post-operative nursing care of stoma patients during appliance changes. Unpublished doctoral dissertation, University of Edinburgh

Green L W 1974 Toward cost benefit evaluations of health education: some concepts methods and examples. Health Education Monographs 2 (supplement): 36–64

Green L W 1977 Evaluation and measurement: some dilemmas for health education. American Journal of Public Health 67 (2): 155–161

Guilbert J J 1977 Educational handbook for health personnel. World Health Organisation Offset Publications No 35 Geneva

Hayward J 1975 Information: a prescription against pain. Royal College of Nursing, London

Rocella E J 1976 Potential for reducing health care costs by public and patient education. Public Health Reports 91 (3): 223–225

FURTHER READING

Abramson J H 1984. Survey methods in community medicine, 3rd edn. Churchill Livingstone, Edinburgh

Tones B K 1977 Effectiveness and efficiency in health education: a review of theory and practice. Scottish Health Education Unit Occasional Paper Scottish Health Education Group, Edinburgh

Treece E W, Treece J W 1977 Elements of research in nursing. 2nd edn. The C V Mosby Company, St Louis

Weiss C H 1978 Evaluating action programmes: reading in social action and education. Allyn and Bacon, Inc. Boston

Knowledge review

1. Which of the following is correct?
   An epidemiologist is concerned with:
   (a) census and registration data   ( )
   (b) collecting data relating to disease   ( )
   (c) examining data to identify contributing   ( )
       factors to disease
   (d) all of the above.   ( )

2. Complete the following statements:
   (a) Statistics which register deaths are called _____
       _____
   (b) The amount of illness in a community is referred to
       as _____
   (c) The Census in Britain has been carried out at 10-
       yearly intervals since 1801 except once when it was
       missed due to _____
   (d) Information collected by the Census provides essen-
       tial background in relation to population size and _
       _____

3. Name 3 types of rate which may be used to examine
   health statistics:
   1 _____ 2 _____ 3 _____

4. Which of the following statements (or combination there-
   of) is the correct response to the sentence below:
   Sir Allen Daley, the Medical Officer of Health for Bootle,
   considered that a Central body for health education was
   needed to:
   (a) co-ordinate efforts
   (b) prevent duplication of effort
   (c) promote health education
   (d) sanction health education efforts and spending.

5. The Cohen Report of 1964 resulted from the investigations
   of which of the following bodies?:
   (a) A Joint Committee of the Central and   ( )
       Scottish Health Services
   (b) The Scottish Council for Health Education   ( )
   (c) The Central Council for Health Education   ( )
   (d) The World Health Organisation.   ( )

6. Discuss how nurses' and patients' views on patients' information needs differ, and the implications of this for
   the nurse's role as health teacher.

7. Discuss the problems for health education policy and/or
   practice inherent in the idea that the purpose of health
   education is to promote health.

8. Discuss the self-care concept and the implications for
   health education.

9. Discuss the proposal that the health educator should not
   manipulate the client.

10. Describe, with reference to a specific example, the edu-
    cational approach to health education. What are its
    limitations?

11. Discuss the advantages and limitations of the media ap-
    proach to health education.

12. Outline an appropriate health education approach for
    each of the following situations:
    (a) The wife of an accountant, who has 2 children at
        home, is about to be discharged 48 hours after de-
        livery of a healthy baby boy.
    (b) A 25-year-old female has had recurrent bouts of cys-
        titis since the age of 12 years. She is asymptomatic
        now, married with no children.

(c) Bus drivers at a local depot have asked the staff of a health education department for information about heart disease. A scare report in a newspaper prompted the enquiry.

13. Label each of the following health teaching situations as centering on one or more of the kinds of learning (cognitive, affective or psychomotor) and explain briefly, why you have so labelled it:

(a) Pre-operative preparation in termination of pregnancy (Label) _____

Explanation:

(b) Diabetic education with an adolescent involved in sport (Label) _____

Explanation:

(c) Self-care education with a person who has a newly-formed stoma (Label) _____

Explanation:

(d) Teaching a group of adolescent girls 'keep fit' exercises (Label) _____

Explanation:

14. Classify the following as:

(a) open-ended questions (b) closed questions (c) leading questions

(i) Can you tell me more about the feelings you have when you meet with friends in a pub? _____

(ii) Where is the pain most severe? _____

(iii) Did you enjoy that film? _____

(iv) Do you find the smell of your colostomy offensive? _____

(v) What is your day like when you are at home? _____

(vi) How long have you felt nervous? _____

(vii) Is the meal delicious? _____

(viii) Where would you like your
smallpox vaccination, the
right arm or the left arm? _____

In the case of leading questions you have identified, make them into open-ended questions.

15. Illustrate how group work techniques might be used in helping young mothers to explore issues of child rearing.

16. Which factors influence the choice of a teaching method or aid?

17. Indicate below which of the following statements (or combinations of statements) about the concept of need are correct:
The concept of need is difficult to discuss because:
(a) it cannot be defined
(b) it has been defined differently by different people
(c) client and professional perceptions of need are the same
(d) it cannot be identified without comprehensive assessment.
 (i) (a) and (b) are correct   ( )
 (ii) (a), (b) and (d) are correct   ( )
(iii) (b) only is correct   ( )
(iv) (b), (c) and (d) are correct   ( )

18. Which of the following learning objectives are stated in terms of observable learner behaviour?

	Yes	No
(a) The purpose of the lesson is to identify the effects of alcohol upon the body.		
(b) As a result of teaching, the learners will understand the effects of alcohol upon the body.		
(c) Learners will be able to understand the effects of alcohol upon the body.		
(d) Learners will fully appreciate the effects of alcohol upon the body.		
(e) Learners will be able to list 4 effects of alcohol upon the body.		

19. Which of the following learning objectives give unambiguous indication of the required standard of performance?

	Yes	No

(a) List 4 effects of alcohol.

(b) Identify psychological and physical effects of alcohol.

(c) Recognise that alcohol has both psychological and physical effects.

(d) Know the percentage of alcohol contained in sherry, whisky, gin, vodka.

(e) Name the percentage of alcohol contained in any 4 different alcoholic drinks.

(f) Name the percentage of alcohol contained in at least 3 out of 4 named alcoholic drinks.

20. Rewrite the following objectives so that they describe terminal behaviour of the learner and indicate unambiguously the criterion of success:
    (a) to know the rules of aseptic technique.
    (b) to feel competent about injecting himself with insulin
    (c) to calculate insulin dosage.

21. Write a set of objectives likely to meet the initial preoperative teaching needs of a 50-year-old woman undergoing hysterectomy for uterine fibroids.

22. Given the following objectives for cognitive learning, outline a suitable lesson plan for a middle-aged man of average intelligence who is leaving hospital to continue drug therapy at home (you may specify the drug).
    Objectives for drug therapy lesson
    As a result of one pre-discharge lesson the person will:
      (i) be able to recognise the drug name on sight
     (ii) pronounce and spell the drug name
    (iii) state the dose to be taken
     (iv) describe when and how the drug should be taken
      (v) list side-effects

23. John McWilliam is 72 years old and due to go home soon. He lives alone, but has an attentive daughter who visits regularly and lives nearby. He has to have three different medications and has become agitated on the two occasions on which his drug regime for home has been discussed. He insists he knows which drugs to take, but

members of the nursing staff are uncertain of this. Draw up a plan for teaching.

24. Ann is six years old, and had a badly injured finger. Surgeons wish to operate, to prevent dysfunction. Her parents reject technological medicine and have refused permission. You have been asked to persuade them to give permission for surgery. What factors will influence your chance of success?

25. Draw up a health teaching assessment form which could be used with a 32-year-old school teacher admitted for laparoscopy for sterilisation purposes. The assessment should include both the need to learn and readiness to learn. Assuming time will be limited (48 hour admission), indicate priorities for teaching.

26. List the information items you consider it would be necessary to present to a woman undergoing cholecystectomy: on admission, prior to theatre, on discharge. What can be done to increase the likelihood that the person receives and remembers the information?

27. List below the ideas about learning which might influence a teaching plan for a 16-year-old male who has to learn how to inject himself with insulin.

28. Discuss the learning difficulties likely to present to a young man with a complicated fracture of the lower leg in respect of the following:
    (a) accomplishing walking with crutches
    (b) understanding the type of surgical procedure performed
    (c) accepting that playing sport can be dangerous
    (d) using a bedpan.

29. Priorise the learning needs of a middle-aged male smoker who suffers from chronic bronchitis and has been admitted to hospital in a very breathless state.

30. Indicate the factors you would consider in planning a demonstration of baby bathing for young mothers.

31. Tick the correct response.
    Evaluation which is done throughout a learning situation is:

(a) summative evaluation ( )
(b) formative evaluation ( )
(c) objective evaluation ( )
(d) learner evaluation. ( )

32. Tick the correct response. ( )
    Evaluation is primarily concerned with:
    (a) assessment of change in the learner's
        health knowledge, behaviour and attitude ( )
    (b) assessing all of the factors influencing
        learning ( )
    (c) those factors in the learning environment
        which affect learning ( )
    (d) learner characteristics which may influence
        learning. ( )

33. A health visitor is evaluating her efforts of teaching new parents about the importance of play in their child's life. Which one or more of the following techniques would be useful in evaluating the process of teaching and learning?
    (a) checklist ( )
    (b) anecdotal notes ( )
    (c) teacher diary ( )
    (d) written assessment. ( )

34. Outline the advantages and limitations of each of the following standards for use in measuring health education outcomes:
    (a) arbitrary standard
    (b) absolute standard
    (c) negotiated standard
    (d) normative standard.

35. Discuss the purposes of planned evaluation of health teaching.

36. Discuss the idea that health education should reduce health care costs.

ANSWERS

1. d
2. (a)—Mortality statistics
   (b)—Morbidity
   (c)—The Second World War
   (d)—Composition
3. 1 Crude; 2 adjusted or standardised; 3 specific
4. a, b and c
5. a
14. (i)–a
    (ii)–c
    (iii)–b
    (iv)–c
    (v)–a
    (vi)–b
    (vii)–c
    (viii)–c
17. b
18. e
19. (a) yes (b) no (c) no (d) yes (e) yes (f) yes
31. b
32. b
33. b and c

Index